Mastering Your Self, Mastering Your World

Living by the Serenity Prayer

Mastering Your Self, Mastering Your World

Living by the Serenity Prayer

John William Reich

PSYCHE BOOKS

Winchester, UK
Washington, USA

First published by Psyche Books, 2015
Psyche Books is an imprint of John Hunt Publishing Ltd., Laurel House, Station Approach,
Alresford, Hants, SO24 9JH, UK
office1@jhpbooks.net
www.johnhuntpublishing.com
www.psyche-books.com

For distributor details and how to order please visit the 'Ordering' section on our website.

Text copyright: John William Reich 2014

ISBN: 978 1 78279 727 2

A CIP catalogue record for this book is available from the British Library.

Design: Lee Nash

Printed and bound by CPI Group (UK) Ltd, Croydon, CR0 4YY

We operate a distinctive and ethical publishing philosophy in
all areas of our business, from our global network of authors to
production and worldwide distribution.

Contents

Acknowledgements

In writing a book that surveys research and clinical practice published in literally thousands of books and articles, the work of a great number of scholars has come to play a major role in this author's ways of thinking about the topic. In some cases, the author has the privilege of meeting and coming to know personally these other scholars. These experiences have been the highlight of my professional career and are gratefully acknowledged. I am hereby stating my deepest appreciation to the following people who have played such a major role in my personal and professional development.

Certainly first and foremost is my wife Deborah Oldfield Reich, a writer, poet, teacher, and above all supportive companion and wife who has uncomplainingly endured my work habits for many years now. Dr. Alex Zautra is the first colleague at Arizona State University who heard me out on the importance of personal mastery and has supported our joint and my single authorship over many publications. Our colleague, Dr. Mary Davis, joined Alex and I in our decades-long collaborations on numerous research projects, grants, and publications covering a wide range of psychological phenomena. A number of our projects, especially the one supporting the research project I presented in Chapter 9, were guided by our Project Director Dr. Maureen Olmsted, and key staff Brendt Parrish and Billie Sandberg. We had the supportive encouragement and intellectual contributions of a number of other researchers whose valuable help it is a pleasure to acknowledge. They are, alphabetically Drs. Glenn Affleck, Frank Infurna, Perry Nicassio, Morris Okun, Anthony Ong, Sanford Roth, Ellen Strand Howard Tennen and William Uttal. In our projects we were fortunate to be joined by successive groups of outstanding graduate students, many of whom are now engaged in their own impressive careers. I

wish to thank, again alphabetically, Anne Arewasikporn, Dr.
Stephanie Brown, Dr. Patrick Finan, Dr. Charles Guarnaccia, Dr.
Sara Gutierres, Dr. Robert Grossman, Dr. Michael McCall, Dr.
Alex Nagurney, Dr. Jason Newsom, Dr. Bruce Smith, Dr. Drew
Sturgeon, and Dr. Jared Younger. Technical help was provided by
Dr. Douglas Kenrick, Ms. Avanna Peeples and Ms. Sara Pennak.
I am most grateful to Dr. Keith Crnic, Chair of the Arizona
State University Department of Psychology, for arranging for
me to have wonderful office space to continue my research and
writing. Finally, the National Institute on Aging supported our
research on various projects: The one most directly related to our
project reviewed in Chapter 9 was: Administrative Supplement,
Resilience and Health in Communities and Individuals (NIH/
NIA R01AG02666006). The photograph of Jeff Lewis presented
in the Introduction was made available by Zachary Velarde.

My wife, friend, and companion Deborah Oldfield Reich has greatly helped me keep a sense of personal mastery during the event-filled development and writing of this book. I can only hope that her own sense of being in control of the events of her life has been enhanced by seeing me through the final completion of this project.

Preface

Given its near-universal popularity, I suspect that you have already read or heard some version of the following "Serenity Prayer" by the American theologian Reinhold Niebuhr:

> *God grant me the serenity*
> *to accept the things I cannot change;*
> *the courage to change the things I can*
> *and wisdom to know the difference.*
> (cited in: http://en.wikiquote.org)

Although these words are only a part of a larger prayer he developed in or around 1943, it is certainly one of the most well-known and often repeated sayings in the English language. It has achieved that renown because it suggests a new angle on how we can deal with our life experiences. His distinction between some "things" and other "things" is indeed more profound and insightful than it may seem at first. As a theologian, he invokes divine intervention to help us achieve the benefits of knowing the difference.

I suggest that there are more earthly forces at work here. I approached Niebuhr's plea to God from a different perspective, a personal mastery perspective, and it is science-based rather than divine-based. I am not proposing that the two approaches are antagonistic, just different. In fact, it is encouraging that there is a deep similarity and overlap of these different views. Since the science I am talking about arose long after 1943, Niebuhr cannot have known about the insights into our well-being that we now have available to us. It is my intent in this book to deal with the same themes that Niebuhr raises but to give you the latest psychological research findings that describe and explain what it means to accept the things that you cannot change, to change those than you can, and to understand the value of knowing the difference.

I believe firmly in the saying, "Knowledge is power." My reason for writing this book is to enhance your empowerment, to give you knowledge, beliefs, and actions that will bring the world of things that Niebuhr mentioned into a new framework for you. I want to give you the same "template" I had when I read his prayer. But my template is based on an impressive array of research studies, all focused on showing us how our physical and mental well-being are intertwined with what we think about ourselves and what we think about the world of events in which we live our lives. The key issue is the extent to which a person believes that they can control the events that they experience, as opposed to experiencing events arising from outside of their personal control. This book summarizes key studies from thousands of research studies extending back over 50 years, studies which consistently show the power of asserting your personal control to achieve goals you desire and accommodating yourself to reality when you cannot. The picture is complex because it involves not only our thoughts about ourselves, but also our thoughts about the way Niebuhr's "things" happen. I want to dissect that complexity and, in doing so, I will show you what a powerful set of principles we now know of the way that the human mind works when it confronts unchangeable things and changeable things. These have a main focus on our human motivation to be master of our lives, to control the events we experience daily, and to feel confident that we can achieve the goals we want and know how to prevent the occurrence of stressful events.

Your own personal mastery beliefs and actual actions to control the events of your life can be enhanced if you choose to accept and adopt as your own the principles I am going to present in this book. They can be the key to your own personal empowerment and resilience as you deal with the events in your life. The final chapter of this book reports on the results of an experimental treatment for enhancing personal mastery beliefs and actions in a sample of community-residing adults. It introduced a technology-based experimental intervention integrating many of the principles of personal control I describe in this book. The results, which I will display in Chapter 9, show graphic evidence of the success of this intervention for improving the mental health and well-being of its participants. You can adopt these principles for your own habits of thought and action for your betterment. They are there for your own personal empowerment.

As you read this book, I want to engage you in what I can call here "interactive reading." I have based the book on a review of rigorous scientific research, revealing basic, fundamental processes which otherwise would be difficult to observe in the routine complexities of our daily living. This approach is reductionistic, revealing the underlying systematic patterns and regularities in our lives. Niebuhr's Serenity Prayer is pitched at another level, but we shall see great similarities and overlaps in the points he is making which are supported by scientific research. But the research goes far beyond his points, and I will be able to (1) show time and time again how far research has come in establishing the terms and conditions of those basic principles, and (2) I will be able to show you how you can adopt those principles into your own lifestyle.

The research principles I will be discussing are just that: General principles, each of which covers a wide range of events and experiences which we all encounter in our daily living. But they are generalized, and at various places in this book I will encourage you to provide your own personal examples, your personal "things" when they are unchangeable and when they are changeable. This is very real and very personal science, and the template and perspective you will develop about your personal mastery as you read these research findings will be developed out of your own unique life circumstances. It will be the foundation of your own sense of personal mastery, the central topic of this research and of this book. But as scientists, we want to be as clear as we can about our subject of study, so in the next chapter, the Introduction, I will unpack and explore the concept of "things," and it is there that we will find the keys to understanding and growing your own personal sense of mastery.

A Note on this book's title, "Mastering Your Self, Mastering Your World"

The title carries a general theme that I will carry throughout this book. When the Serenity Prayer draws the distinction between the things that you can change and those that you cannot, and the wisdom to know the difference, I am suggesting that you can accept that critical distinction into your own life. I present numerous compelling studies to make it real for you. If you personally accept it, it will become a bedrock set of beliefs and actions and these will empower you to "master your self." The second half of the title follows from the same distinction, but it emphasizes that there is a world of events outside of you, and it is equally important that you learn that some events in your world will not, cannot, and will never respond to your mastery beliefs and actions. It is the greatest part of empowerment to "know the difference," and as a fully functioning person you can make your understanding of that difference your key to mastering your world as well as yourself. That is why I have written this book, and I am eager to join forces with you to help you achieve all that you can be.

Introduction

First, let me start to challenge you with a question. What makes you happy? If you could have a wish granted that would make you as happy as you could want to be, what is that wish? A lot of human history is written in the answers that people give to it.

But before you come up with a quick, off-the-cuff answer, I suggest that you be careful: This is not a trick question, but it is a tricky question, and it is a tricky question for a number of important reasons. I have written this book to help you to see the complications in trying to get an answer to it. You can learn a lot if you will bear with me as we unpack the question. It is going to take a book's worth of discussion to provide the outlines for an answer to it. And it will have to be *your* answer. The one sure source of your empowerment in your life is you.

In this book I will present information about a number of scientifically-established principles of how we achieve happiness. But at the same time, I assume that you would also want to avoid unhappiness, and those same principles show where such unhappy conditions as sadness and depression come from and can be avoided. Since these principles are based on deeply-embedded psychological processes in your personality and in the ways you respond to your environment, only you can adapt those principles and make them fit who you are. Although we all want to be happy, whatever that means, happiness does not mean being competent or in control of the events of your life. In fact, it may be a fundamental misdirection away from achieving more fundamental strengths and capacities which can enhance your empowerment and resilience as you encounter stresses and challenges in your life. At the end of this chapter I will raise a caution about this issue of "being happy," suggesting that we focus instead on the principles of personal mastery and competence at achieving our goals. And I discuss this issue in more detail in Chapter 5 where I deal with the role of desirable events in our well-being.

The key to these principles resides in the realm of what therapists and researchers call, with varying terms, "personal causation." I gave you a brief summary of this concept with the term "personal mastery" in my Preface, and I will discuss other terms and meanings in later chapters. This general term refers to the beliefs and actions when people come to assert control over the events of their lives. So in this book I will deal extensively with how you exercise your freedom of choice as you go about the activities of your daily living. With those principles explained and with numerous examples I will provide to make them real for your own thinking, the second half of this book will give you some proven laboratory-tested and field-tested guidelines for using those principles to manage your own life to achieve better happiness, however you define it.

The following simple example will give you a quick demonstration of some of the complications involved in the question about how to achieve happiness. Listed below are two columns of very common, daily events that occur in the lives of nearly everyone. Look over the lists and think about each event as if it has occurred in your life. In terms of your happiness, which ones would you want to happen, and which ones would you not want to happen?

Column A (1st listing)	Column B (1st listing)
You went to a movie	You drove dangerously in traffic
You helped someone out	A good friend contacted you
Someone was critical of you	You started an argument
You were insensitive to someone	Someone smiled nicely at you
You bought some ice cream	You got the flu
Someone told you something amazing	You had a flat tire

I know that these are very different events, but they are common occurrences and some of them may have occurred in your life recently. But before you make your final choice, I want to rearrange them into a different pair of categories. You will you see the same events but this re-grouping is different. It may now be obvious that I initially listed them above in a random order, but this new order is not at all random. The difference from the first listing will make a difference in your life. See if you can detect the organizing principle behind the new listing. Again, I will list the events in two columns, but this time the columns should have a different meaning for you.

New Column A (2nd listing)	New Column B (2nd listing)
You went to a movie	You drove dangerously in traffic
You helped someone out	You were insensitive to someone
A good friend contacted you	Someone was critical of you
You bought some ice cream	You started an argument
Someone smiled nicely at you	You got the flu
Someone told you something amazing	You had a flat tire

It should be pretty obvious that Column A is a list of generally positive, favorable, nice-when-it-happens daily events. We would all like them to happen more often, and more events of this generally positive type would be welcome any time. But the events listed in Column B are not at all favorable, and most of us would rather not have such undesirable events happen in our lives.

However, if you are a careful reader, you might feel that you have yet a different take on those events. Even though it is clear why I have grouped them into List A's desirable events and List B's undesirable events, you may well have seen another principle that could have been used to group them. Again, this difference makes a difference. Let me step in here and recategorize these same 12 events all over again, again using two columns but this time the new columns are based on an entirely different categorizing principle:

New Column A (3rd listing)	**New Column B (3rd listing)**
You bought some ice cream	A good friend contacted you
You went to a movie	Someone told you something amazing
You were insensitive to someone	Someone smiled nicely at you
You drove dangerously in traffic	You got the flu
You helped someone out	You had a flat tire
You started an argument	Someone was critical of you

As you can tell, categorizing events this way mixes up the desirable or undesirable distinction, but now I have separated them into a category of those events which you personally could have made happen, ones which you caused to occur (Column A): Your own *personal control* over making those events occur is their real cause. But Column B regroups them as events that happen to you without you making any effort or exercising personal control over them. Events in this list are events that occurred separately from your own actions and, in the language I will be using in this book, they are "uncontrollable" events. But now they may not have the same positive/negative tone: Some of them are desirable which you made occur and some are negative which you made occur, so their positive/negative tone may not be as important to you as whether or not you had personal control over their occurrence. This makes judging them a more complicated process than it may have appeared. As I said earlier, asking you what makes you happy is not a trick question, but answering it can indeed be tricky.

Categorizing everyday events in these distinctly different ways allows us to determine the *causal nature* of the event and how that principle of event causation relates to who we are and how we manage our lives. The larger question is, which category of event occurrence has the greatest positive or negative impact on our mental and even our physical health? Now you can see why I said in the Preface that Reinhold Niebuhr's term "things" was complex. If you want to really do something with the Serenity Prayer, if you want to see how it fits your own life, then a lot more needs to be said about it. Research has revealed principles of our mental health and well-being that show how to unpack the concept of "things" so that we can apply the Prayer to our own lives.

With this more complex but more sophisticated approach to exactly what is involved with each and every event that happens in our lives, researchers and practitioners have been able to ask a series of questions such as these:

Is it better to arrange your life so that you cause only positive events to occur in your life (as much as possible, anyway?) Or,

Is it better for you to make sure that you do not cause any undesirable events to occur in your life (as much as possible, anyway)? Or,

Is it better to have a life in which you personally make both desirable and undesirable events happen in your life (as much as possible, anyway?), Or,

Is it better to have a life in which you do not control either desirable or undesirable events to occur, a life in which things are done for you (at least, as much as possible, anyway)?

Of course, we could mix-and-match these combinations up to a large number of alternatives, too many to list here. This is a very rich way of thinking about our lives, and it has been very productive for researchers and mental and physical health practitioners. Many subtle aspects of the ways we live our lives become clearer when we understand the complications of how all of these parts are interconnected. Even better, this way of thinking suggests clinical interventions to improve people's happiness and well-being. For instance, now we can ask, is it better to have a person spend their personal energies trying to increase the number of desirable events in their lives? That would be fine, except that it is inevitably the case that some desirable events come from the actions of other people; and those would be externally-caused, "out of your control" events. We would need to understand the research findings on the effects of externally-caused events before we could answer this question.

The other side of that coin is, should we encourage people to be active causes of the events of their lives, both desirable and undesirable, and avoid situations where they are exposed to events outside of their control? But encouraging people to avoid out-of-personal-control events means that they may not seek help from valuable external sources of aid; reliance on others as caregivers, as providers of resources for our own well-being is often a wise course of action. On the other hand, actively thinking that you are the cause of undesirable events can have positive effects on your mental health. As implausible as that may seem, I will research findings which show that to be the case.

These question are important to explore both for you as an individual person and for society in general. How much should we "help" people? Can we build a society in which people experience only undeviatingly positive experiences? Can we build a society in which people are protected from harmful experiences by giving up their personal control to external sources of control? By reviewing a number of research studies and understanding the principles of how events relate to mental and physical health, we can start to frame these questions in ways that can be helpful for you the individual and the broader society that we have created for ourselves.

Neutral Events, Neither Positive nor Negative

So far, my discussion of events has been rather lopsided: I have only talked about desirable and undesirable events. Even at that, you can see that it is a complicated issue. But now let me suggest to you yet another set of events that do not appear in our lists above. Think about them as if they have occurred recently in your life.

Column A (4th listing)   **Column B (4th listing)**
You drove/biked to work   Someone started a conversation
You picked up your   It rained on your lawn
  newspaper
You turned on your radio/TV   Someone told you a news item

These are pretty mundane items, and you could easily list a dozen more without thinking very hard about them, and in fact such mundane events may well outnumber the more colorful desirable and undesirable events just in frequency alone. Being so common, then we have to factor them into our equation about how to understand happiness and unhappiness. What is the difference? These events are neutral in tone, moderate, they are not particularly evaluative and they do not elicit particularly strong emotional feelings from you one way or other. Are they not worth discussing? While they are neutral in content, they are nevertheless good examples of personally-caused events (in Column A), and the events in Column B are caused by forces outside of you, either the weather (over which of course we have no control) or they are caused by other people, again without our own personal causation. This gives them great psychological significance even though they may initially seem routine and not very interesting; but in fact they are very interesting, as you will see as I probe more deeply into events and personal mastery.

So these items show that we should distinctly separate out from events their positive/negative emotional loading from their personal internal/external causation loading. Studying neutral or moderate events does this for us neatly: They are very frequent but by separating out their "locus of causation" they help us look at issues of event control processes separately from any emotional loadings they may have. Here, then, we can get relatively pure tests of personal control in and of itself.

This is a key consideration for scientists and they explore the processes and outcomes of personal causation, *per se,* from the positive or negative reactions we experience when we, or someone or something else, leads us to have experiences outside of our personal control. As we review the research studies and therapies in this book, separating these control-based components of our overall mental and physical health has to involve learning how we can best develop and apply our own personal control beliefs and actions.

Major Events also "Happen"

There is another layer of complication that now arises. Those small daily events are only a part of our lives: Major, heavy-impact events also arise in our lives, some caused by us and some caused by forces outside of us. For instance, "getting married" or "getting a new job" or "retiring from work" are certainly major events (ones we caused) and "being laid off" or "having a serious accident" or "developing a chronic painful illness" are also major events, in this case caused by forces outside of us. Such events are of course much less common than the mundane events of our daily life, but because of their magnitude, they can become more impactful, positively or negatively, on our mental health and well-being. How do they fit into the picture of how we can use these principles of event causation to enhance our capacities for managing our lives?

Events in the Life of Jeff Lewis of Mesa, Arizona

To introduce you to this important area of research on factors contributing to our well-being, a story involving one such event will give you a flavor of how important, but again how tricky, it is to ask the question if someone is "happy."

I want to describe here the nature of "major life events" by relaying to you the story of a Mesa, Arizona man, Mr. Jeff Lewis. His story was published in the Dec. 8, 2010 issue of the *Arizona Republic* newspaper. Jeff's story began when he merely happened to be standing in the backyard of his Mesa home one day when the teenage boy next door got into his parents' gun cabinet. The boy took the loaded gun into his family's backyard and began firing it. A bullet went through the fence and hit Jeff in the back, destroying his spleen. Medical help was available and he was rushed to the hospital for immediate treatment. As you might expect, surgery was required and fortunately it was successful. He recovered from the surgery and returned to his work as a Mesa high school teacher for the next two years, at which time he retired from his teaching career.

However, his body's natural defenses against infection had become compromised by the bullet and the surgery. In retirement, he contracted a staph infection and, with no functioning immunity, he physically collapsed and nearly died. Again in the hospital, surgeons found the damage from the infection to be so severe that the only way he could survive was to have his extremities, both hands and both feet, surgically removed. He did survive again and bounced back once more, displaying to my mind extraordinary resilience.

But there is more to his story. Jeff then faced life as a paraplegic. But he quickly became bored with his new condition. Striving for greater happiness in his life, he approached local prosthesis manufacturers with a plan to fit him out with artificial arms and legs. They did so successfully, and Jeff then began to learn how to return to the good parts of his former life. A picture of Jeff enjoying his new style of life tells much of the story.

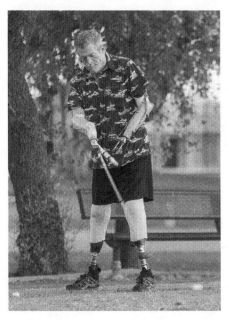

Jeff Lewis Enjoying Golf, His Favorite Pasttime

As you can see, he is playing golf! That is not new because he was an avid golfer before the accident (although that does not make it any less amazing!). But that is only part of his new life. He is now an avid dancer, he puts in many hours of volunteer work counseling other patients, and he gives public talks about his experiences. (If you want to learn more about him, here is his website address: *http://www.dontworryaboutme.com*.) His personal motto says it all: "Don't let what you can't do get in the way of what you can do."

Jeff Lewis's story is rich in so many ways: Psychologists would say that his reactions involved cognitive, emotional, motivational processes. (1), *Cognitive,* because his thoughts about his disability drove him to find new ways to think about himself and to think about new ways to go about living his life again; (2), *Emotional,* in that he responded to his accident with a pattern of positive feelings about his chances for recovery, rather than negative thoughts such as depression and withdrawal; and (3), *Motivational,* in that he moved forward from the original experience and engaged his high level of drive to be active and to restore his control over the events of his daily life.

Having all three of these psychological processes wrapped up in one experience is truly remarkable. All of these in one way or another engage important psychological processes as we navigate through the good times and bad times of our lives. But I want to argue that there is an even deeper level of meaning underlying his story, and it is important for all of us to grasp the significance of what he has done.

A review of the psychological research literature would have easily led to a very clear prediction about how Jeff *should have* ended up after his surgery, a very different prediction than what actually occurred. Since the "accident" was really an externally-caused undesirable event, research says that he should have become dominated by negative emotions. There are two reasons for that prediction. One, because the experience was negative (my second column of event listings in my examples above) and, two, because it was an externally-caused event (my third set of event listings above). On solid research grounds, then, we would have predicted that he would become depressed, that he would experience "learned helplessness" (described later in Chapter 4), and he would have been expected to withdraw socially and perhaps he might even have entertained suicidal thoughts. But these reactions did not occur, nowhere near to his real reactions. I want to ask why they did not.

To begin, let's go back over the Jeff Lewis experience, this time taking an entirely different approach to it. Let me list some new ways to think about his story.

1. The first question we might want to ask it, *why* do we find ourselves feeling amazement here in this story (and of course, admiration)? Why would we expect him *not* to cope so well? We would naturally expect him to be psychologically wiped out, withdrawn, perhaps suicidal, and at the very least in a state of "giving up." Since he clearly is not depressed, negative, or withdrawn, then we are justified in being amazed. But are we correct in assuming those negative, maladaptive states should invariably occur when a major undesirable externally-caused event happens to someone? What is it about such terrible experiences that make us expect the worst, rather than seeing the possibilities for recovery, sustainability, and growth? Perhaps we should rethink the impact of undesirable experiences on people, even a severe one such as Jeff experienced.

2. What is about an *accident,* per se, that makes it so destructive, as opposed to some mistake we ourselves make. Certainly Jeff did nothing to make this happen... an entirely external cause of the event is what brought it about. Is there a difference between self-caused events as opposed to those events that just happen, that arise from external causes? Why would this distinction between internally-caused events and externally-caused events be an important distinction? Earlier, I have provided you with examples of daily events which vary in causation. So now we have to see that distinction pay off in getting a better understanding of the optimum ways to live your life.

3. Why are undesirable events so much more impactful than desirable ones? Since I am claiming that the nature of the

event causation, internal *vs.* external is so important, then that by itself would logically suggest that if some externally-caused desirable event had happened, then that should have an equally destructive impact on someone experiencing it. To find a comparable example, suppose Jeff had been in his backyard and got a notice that he had just won a lottery with a big amount of money? That is a classic example of "externally-caused but this time desirable event." Why would we expect this not to have a destructive negative impact on him, since it was an externally-caused event? Clearly we would not expect winning a lottery to have bad consequences on a person. After all, that is why people gamble their money, in fact often losing but coming back for more. (Again, this is not a trick question, but it is a tricky question; See Chapter 5).

Research shows that desirable events and positive emotions have the effect of opening up our mind and creating new thoughts and behaviors, while negative events shut us down and make us withdraw.[1] And perhaps most interesting of all, results of psychological studies on lottery winners show that they may feel less anxiety and depression but their immediate reactions show that they are *not* happier than the rest of us. In fact, one study shows that they rate the quality of their lives as poorer and more unpleasant than us non-winners. Would you really like a life in which you had to do nothing at all but experience desirable events? Again, that may sound implausible to you right now, but the research shows it to be not only plausible, but quite understandable given the way the mind works. Clearly there is a lot of information that people need to know about the important principles of the differences between undesirable and desirable experiences simply from knowing what caused them to occur.

4. What if Jeff's attempts to get his life back into some semblance of his former life had *not* actually worked? What would have been the consequences if he failed to gain control of his life? What happens to us if we try to make something happen, to create a new set of conditions and experiences for ourselves, but we find that we have failed in the attempt? What if we try to get control and mastery over our daily living, but are thwarted and blocked in our attempts? Research shows this failure of attempts at control to have serious "cognitive, emotional, and motivational" consequences. Some environments are deliberately arranged so that the individual cannot get control and cannot exercise their sense of personal mastery: Prisons, hospitals, and the military are social institutions where the individual is not supposed to be in control of their lives. What about nursing homes where the staff is trained to make the residents rely on them, the staff, rather than going off on their own? Should teachers allow students a free environment where the teacher exercises no classroom control? These examples demonstrate the important differences in the *process* of control attempts, as much as it shows the importance of the *outcome* of the process.

The overarching principle in the Jeff Lewis story is that he took personal control of his fate, he exercised his beliefs in his own personal mastery, he took control over the development of his prostheses, and he is now in control of his daily activities and his public engagements. His "disorder," the original medical problem and his follow-up condition is not controlling his life. Jeff Lewis is. I would argue that taking control over his life's events has led him to be highly resilient in the face of what many of us would probably consider a personal disaster.

Without further investigation we do not know exactly which aspect of his life was engaged so successfully: It could be his background childhood experiences, it could be his genetics, and it very well could be part of his personality traits and stable, enduring beliefs in his own personal mastery. Shortly I will discuss the many versions of research techniques which have been developed to measure "belief in personal control" and he may well have scored highly on those tests. But with just the story we now have, there is no sure way of finding out about those hidden possible causes. But what we do know is that his story is an outstanding example of a person demonstrating the power of personal control over the events of his life.

My colleagues Alex Zautra, Mary Davis, and John Hall and our many allied colleagues consider Jeff Lewis's story to be a premier example of what has come to be called in the social sciences, a story of *resilience*. You can read about this approach on our website, http://www.asu.edu/resilience. We define adult resilience to mean the ability to rebound (R) from a stressor, to sustain (S) that response, and to grow (G) from the experience. Thus we have named our interdisciplinary team the Arizona State University Resilience Solutions Group (RSG), to capture the essence of exactly the experience that Jeff Lewis has demonstrated. We consider personal control to be a key to resilient response under stress. A number of disciplines are represented in this new approach to well-being, many of which are summarized in our book, *Handbook of Adult Resilience.*[2] We have published some of our findings in a recent technical paper in which we present the core components of the actual experimental manipulation that I present in the second half of this book.[3]

I started out this book with Reinhold Niebuhr's Serenity Prayer which has, at its core meaning, the very ambiguous concept of "things." I am replacing it with the term "events," and you can now see how more complex but more realistic for your own life the personal mastery approach can be.

An Overview of the Contents of this Book
Now I want to give you a brief overview of how this book
is organized. In the first half of this book I will lay out the
particulars of how you experience life's events, big and small,
desirable and undesirable, controllable and not controllable.
The nature of personal causation or external causation of those
events is the key. Once that is understood in all of its "trickiness,"
then you are closer to seeing how your own personal cognitive,
emotional, and motivational powers and capacities can be
marshaled for you to optimize your well-being. Understanding
how these mental forces intertwine will help you employ beliefs
in your own personal mastery demonstrating how you can
reshape your ways of thinking about life's events. My intent is
for you to understand when you can control those events and
when those events are out of your control and how you can
respond well even then. Jeff Lewis did.

Following the basic research on many aspects of control,
beliefs and actions, covered in Chapters 2 through 5, I will then
discuss in Chapter 6 some actual experimental interventions and
techniques which therapists and researchers have developed to
help people enhance their sense of mastery over the events of
their lives. I will describe a number of experimentally-tested
techniques for enhancing personal control so that you can see
the ways in which personal beliefs can match personal capacities
with the controllable and uncontrollable events of your life.
These techniques rest on solid foundations of concepts and
theories of personal mastery which I will have presented earlier
so you will have the best available evidence of the power of this
way of thinking.

Chapter 7 reviews the previous chapters' findings from
research studies and extracts from them nine major conclusions
about what that research is saying about how personal mastery
functions for a person in their environment of events. These
conclusions represent general principles of how personal

mastery influences mental health and well-being. Chapter 8 then displays two general categorical schemes which present, graphically, how the personal control approach organizes the many different facets of personal control perspective on events and their properties. One major category system organizes events into their properties of controllability and how those properties distinguish categories of our life events (Figure 8.1). At the end of the chapter, a graphic display of how a person's core beliefs in their own personal mastery relate to their environment of controllable and uncontrollable events (Fig. 8.2).

Following the presentation of the many ways in which personal mastery connects with the major and small events of our lives and our mental and physical health, in the last chapter of this book I will present a thorough description of the experimental study and instructions which my colleagues Alex Zautra, Mary Davis and I employed to enhance the personal mastery beliefs and actions of our adult research participants. Our experimental test of the effectiveness of this intervention showed that it had significantly favorable outcomes. You yourself can use them to empower yourself to gain greater mastery of the events in your own life. You can develop your own personal mastery template to guide your understanding of the world in which you live. And with the very same template, you can gain a better understanding of other people's worlds and the way their personal mastery functions for them. After all, *you* are an event, desirable or undesirable, in their lives, and knowing that may have beneficial effects on the ways you understand and appreciate them.

No, I Am Not Trying to Make You Happier

Now that I have given you the general points of the personal mastery approach to mental health and well-being, this is the appropriate time to make what appears to be an outrageous claim. In spite of what I said earlier, in fact I emphatically do *not* have the intent to make you happy. I began this chapter by having you think about ways you can be happy and the kinds of events that can get you there. But the material I will discuss in this book should have you rethink having happiness as the single most important goal of your life.

I have several reasons for saying this. First, I have no idea what you personally find to be your best route to finding happiness. I can be certain that different readers have different ideas of happiness, and it would be fruitless for me to try to connect with every reader's particular goals for attaining it. Second, I would caution you to "be careful what you wish for." What might at first appear to be a desirable experience can have a significant downside to it, as we shall see in Chapter 5. In her recent book, *The Myths of Happiness: What should make you happy, but doesn't; What shouldn't make you happy, but does,* Sonja Lyubomirksy[4] presents compelling evidence that our commonsense ways of thinking about happiness are often wrong. Further, what might be initially a negative or stressful experience can have benefits above and beyond any momentary happiness one might feel. And you could be wrong about what you guess will make you happy. In his revealing book, *Stumbling on Happiness5*, Daniel Gilbert[5] has amassed convincing research evidence that we are terrible at predicting what will make us happy. We simply cannot have the evidence now at hand to predict what our actual feelings will be when we attain what we think will make us happy. Third, there is good reason to say that if you can achieve whatever it is that makes you happy, there still is no guarantee that you will be taking care of things that make you unhappy. As surprising as this may seem, there is little reason to assume that happiness and unhappiness are just automatically hooked to each other, such that changing one will automatically change the other. "Going to a movie" when you want to be happy is likely to make you happier, but going to a movie to overcome the anger and frustration of "a fight with a loved one" is not likely to remove that anger and frustration. This is partly a logical matter, but there is a good deal of psychological research showing that in fact we have two separate emotional systems, positive and negative (for a short-cut label), not one system with two opposite ends. It would deflect me from my main point of this book to get into this big body of research, but I can refer you to one article I have published which reviews a good deal of that research.[6]

With the assumption that this book's material can make you "happy" out of the way, what I *can* propose is to give you the research concepts, theories, and especially findings of studies which can enhance your sense of personal mastery over the events of your life. I can claim the goal of giving you ways to (1) pursue desirable events that you want to happen in your life and (2) to find ways to deal effectively with undesirable events in your life. I believe that resilience and empowerment are keys to a better life, if not a happier one, and both of these outcomes result from a greater sense of personal control over life's experiences.

Many years ago in a now classic article, the psychologist Robert White[7] redirected our notions of human motivation as being based solely on biological drives. We are much more than that narrow view suggests: He argues that we strive for competence, which he defined as "...an organism's capacity to interact effectively with the environment" (1959, p. 297). Competence is a key indicator of heightened personal mastery, and "effective interacting" is a much more powerful indicator of successful mental health than the fleeting pursuit of "happiness" whatever it might be.

The bottom line of the perspective I am presenting in this book is that control over the events of your life is a key to successful living in obtaining desirable events and avoiding undesirable ones. If I have one success in writing this book and if you have one success in reading it, that success is not measured in "happiness units" whatever they might be, but that you find greater success in these two main goals of an effective life.

A Note on Research and, Especially, Statistics

The issues I have raised in this chapter and their possible answers are tricky. I am saying that they are tricky because both the questions and their answers are complex and subtle. But they are *not* unanswerable. In fact, research on positive and negative life experiences and the conditions and situations of personal control and mastery are one of the largest topics of research in all of the social sciences, particularly experimental, clinical, and social psychology. There is a huge storehouse of solid, empirically-validated studies on a whole range of these issues. The problem is that this research, as rich and as useful as it is, is archived in technical journals, reports, and books, and this work is almost completely unknown to the general public. Professionals in many areas know of it and employ it in their technical work, but the public is where the science could have its greatest impact, both on individuals and on social policy. In that spirit, therefore, I have written this book not for technical professionals but for you personally and for the public at large where, I believe, it can do the most good.

This book is a review and summary of a large body of research in the social sciences, particularly psychology, the science of the individual person. To do that, I am taking what is a frankly "reductionist" approach; I will deal with what research says about basic, fundamental, and elementary processes, with facts, that are solidly based on research findings. What I will be discussing here is almost entirely based on quantitative analyses of samples of individuals who have responded in some way to provide information on their thoughts about their lives and the events that they have been experiencing. My assumption as a scientist is that the responses of that sample will be typical of any individual in the group. That is pretty much the way any science works: Find the general tendency, the average response, and that will be the best predictor of any particular member of that sample being tested. Of course, with human beings, this becomes complex: We are all different in so many ways. But while the general average may miss being exactly true of any particular individual such as you, it is still the best overall predictor. So I am presenting the results of these studies assuming that they will apply more closely to you personally, better than any other measure. I hope that you will find these many results at least reasonably close to your own experiences, thoughts, and feelings about your life. That is why I have stated in the Preface that you will gain the most if you engage in "interactive reading" as you read through the many studies and their results that are highlights of the personal mastery approach.

And let me add that I have gone lightly over the actual statistical methods used by these experimenters. I will avoid burying you in details of methods and numbers; this is a book about ideas and how you can use them, and I've left the details up to the specialists. I'm giving you the music, not the notes: I hope that you enjoy the performance.

Chapter 1

Paying Attention to Your Daily Events

To begin, let me make a prediction about people, including you and me, and see if you agree with me. Suppose that we take a randomly-selected person and observe that person for a 24-hour period of their daily living. Subtracting out their sleeping time when they are not deliberately active, what guess would you make about what they will be doing during that time?

Although they might at first appear to be doing seemingly different and varied things during the day, I predict that they will be engaging in two general classes of actions that will be easily observable to all of us. I am pretty sure that in any ordinary day, any person will be: (1) trying to get the things they want and (2) they will be trying to avoid things that they do not want. I will predict the same for you and for me as well. It is indeed a simple interpretation of our behavior, and I am guessing that you may think it is too simple. Surely there is more to us than that. But even if it were a true picture of our personal daily actions, I will argue in this book that it would still only be half of the story. It focuses too much on the individual person as an active, independent entity and it does not say enough about the external world where we conduct our lives. Focusing just on the person has the rather perverse effect of leading us to ignore that person's environment, where a continuous blizzard of events is always in action. This external environment which we call "reality" has a way of intruding in our lives, and our success at pursuing these two goals is sometimes helped and sometimes hindered by the world in which we live. I hope that you would join me in wanting to help you achieve both types of goals. That was my reason for writing this book.

The Goal of Self-Actualization

Social science research has learned a lot about how we strive to achieve a satisfying life by pursing those two general goals, actually more than you might suspect. While much of this groundbreaking work is stored away in technical journals, my aim here is to collect systematically those research findings in this one book and to bring them to your attention in nontechnical language (as much as possible). My career-long premise is that social science research is highly relevant to the individual person, you and me, and it can help everyone improve their lives. It is my statement of faith that you can adopt as your own the principles of human happiness (both types) presented in this book and in doing so you will find your own personal paths to your goals more open and effective for you.

Human society has evolved many varieties of individual, family, and societal structures to foster our quests for a better life. Nearly every aspect of human social organization in one way or another has been developed to support what is basically a human motivation for *self-actualization*, to use rather academic language coined by Abraham Maslow.[1] He meant that we are motivated for action to fulfill all of our potential. You can think of this "self-ish" motivation as a master motive to be all that we can be.

But of course this self-ishness is not the only engine driving our life. Helping others actualize their own capacities is nearly equally dominant in human social consciousness. We strive to help our children, our family, our acquaintances and even total strangers to achieve their maximum potential as well. There are many examples of entities we have created to help people grow their strengths and conquer their weaknesses. The examples of these social entities are everywhere around us in our environment: Education, healthcare, charity, and even government itself are all mechanisms we develop to make sure that people get what they need to achieve their maximum potential. We can call this second process "other-actualization" for want of a neater term.

One important value of the personal mastery approach to life is that, even in the face of a lot of uncontrollable events which might occur in your experiences, your *belief* in your own personal mastery can still be intact. Every day we see instances of how people respond to undesirable events by bouncing back, by steadfastly continuing to cope while attempting to keep their lives livable and forward-moving. One is reminded of this repeatedly when television and radio news presents scenes of natural and man-made disasters, some of which may have happened to you or your loved ones. But note that we also discover in these situations people immediately looking to rebuild, to bounce back, to move forward. This is human resilience, one of the demonstrations of what psychologist Anne Masten[2] has called "ordinary magic." This magic is, in fact, almost routine in the face of the many kinds of disasters that we see repeatedly in our local and national newscasts. From the personal mastery perspective, I would argue that, even though the material possessions of these people may have been damaged or even destroyed, nevertheless their *beliefs* are still their own, protected, and enduring possessions in spite of everything external that may occur. Humans are almost infinitely adaptable, they are naturally resilient in the face of disasters, and their beliefs are what can sustain them in otherwise devastating circumstances. Being prepared by being aware of the causal contours of your world is your best hope for recovery and growth. Understanding the causes of events is a key to being prepared for your most effective adaptation.

In this book I am going to present some fundamental principles of happiness and sadness which research in psychology and the social sciences have found to be key components of resilience, growth, and self-actualization. This body of discoveries has revealed the critical links between a person's inner drives for actualizing their capacities and the external world in which they live. In contemporary terms, the concept that captures the essence of this linking of both worlds is "empowerment." There seems to be a good deal of controversy over the best definition of the term, but by a computer search I located two sources and definitions that best fit the model of actualization I am developing in this book:

> *empowerment... to give someone more control over their life or more power to do something... make stronger and more confident, especially in controlling their life and claiming their rights*
> http://www.macmillandictionary.com

Control Over What?

To apply basic principles of control to our quest for empowerment, we first have to ask, "Control over *what*"? If you are to achieve empowerment, what would you *do*? How would it show up in your daily life? Would you know that you have gained the correct amount of empowerment, or how would you know that you need more treatment?

There are many angles to consider in answering these questions, but in this book I propose that there are certain *fundamental* ways of thinking and action in your life that can give you a distinct, focused, and clear sense of the conditions necessary to your empowerment. Many of the components of empowerment thinking have some features in common with the social programs and structures that I mentioned above. But what I am presenting to you here is a unique approach. It is based on psychological research, it has proven validity and it is realistic, in the sense that it is based on the experiences of people dealing with the events of their daily living as you and I do. I want to help you "scaffold" your thinking and actions in your life onto a foundation of established research findings about the factors involved in what actually relates to enhanced well-being.

But the approach I am presenting here in this book takes a hard turn away from the theme of empowerment in one crucial way. As I said in this chapter's opening paragraph, life is not simple; it is complicated and the paths to our goals are often difficult to follow. Sometimes any sense of empowerment must face the inevitable fact that much of our life takes place outside our own sphere of empowerment. Things happen in the world outside of us, and these things impinge on us, sometimes supporting our goal-strivings and sometimes hindering them. The most important characteristic that we need to understand is that these things sometimes happen beyond your own personal control. Some of these are desirable, some are more undesirable, and some are more neutral in tone, but in all cases for this category of life experiences, we have nothing to do with their occurrence. Yet when they enter our life, they can either support or challenge any sense of empowerment that we may have developed.

This is a crucial distinction: Some of our life's events arise because we want them to occur or we find ways to avoid them; this is the essence of empowerment. But you cannot control an earthquake, a tornado, or a nice present that someone might give you unexpectedly, "out of the blue," or a layoff notice from your employer. What does an empowerment way of thinking say about such externally-caused events? If this book is going to help you gain empowerment, if it is going to "...give someone more control over their life or more power to do something" as the definition says, then we have to clarify this key difference in internal *vs.* external causes of the events that you experience in your life.

To fully apply this distinction in our own lives while keeping in the spirit of Reinhold Niebuhr's Serenity Prayer requires that we move to a different approach to his concept of "things."

To do that I want to unpack the meaning of the concept of "event." This is where I will differ from standard treatments of empowerment. This seemingly simple concept defines the realities of our lives as we pursue our goals. It encapsulates your actions and reactions that establish and maintain your empowerment, and it is the most important concept I am using in this book. Again, I will turn to a standard dictionary definition to establish what it is I am going to present in this book:

> *event... something that takes place, an occurrence*
> (http://www.thefreedictionary.com)

Something so seemingly simple as the concept of events or occurrence may not immediately strike you as particularly crucial for your empowerment. Eating your breakfast is an event. Washing your dishes is an event. Dating someone is an event. So is getting a divorce, as is getting married. Events are everywhere everyday all of our lives. They are so common that at first glance it may seem that there cannot be anything very interesting about them. However, literally hundreds of psychological research studies have now accumulated enough information that we can now consider focusing on our events to be a major key to understand how life actually occurs on a daily basis. Thinking of events as signals important to your mental and physical health, and to your empowerment, may strike you as unusual and perhaps a bit mysterious. But the research I will discuss in this book repeatedly shows how an event-focused approach gives very useful insights into some of the major influences on your well-being.

Let Us Unpack the Concept of "Event"

I am suggesting that you take what might strike you as an unfamiliar view of your life, an event-based view. You are certainly fully aware of the individual, discrete experiences of the events of your life as you live them on a daily basis. But now I am suggesting that you move up one level of awareness and adopt a framework, an overall structure, into which you can fit your experiences, organizing them and systematically understanding the similarities and differences that give each event its unique properties, positive or negative (it works both ways, and that is its strength). It will help you greatly when you become aware of the critical *properties* of each event which research has shown gives us insights into their power and influence over how we live our lives. That structure or framework for understanding events reveals four major properties: Their *magnitude,* their *emotional valen*ce, their one-time-only or chronic *recurrence* and, most importantly from the perspective of this book, the extent to which you can or cannot *control* their occurrence.

I will discuss each of these event properties next. To describe them, I will make quick points and short descriptions to give you a beginning idea of what each property is in practice. I describe those event properties in more detail beginning in Chapter 3 and then follow up on those principles in subsequent chapters.

Events are discrete occurrences. Events are experiences which have a beginning, a duration, and they may or may not have a discrete ending. Once they occur, they have the effect of exerting some form of pressure, positive or negative, to do something about them. They draw us to them because they are desirable, or they threaten our well-being because they are undesirable. Even neutral events such as going to the grocery store puts some pressure on us to "get it done." They have implications for our thoughts, feelings, and our actions. But they are not necessarily a single-occurrence; some may occur over and over, and they vary in chronicity... some end cleanly like washing your dishes, others have a lingering duration such as getting married. They are the kinds of experiences that fill up our day, they are what we tell other people when they ask, "Hey, what's going on?" They are what we ask other people about when we talk with them. Of course events happen to other people, but in my approach I want to deal just with events that arise in your own personal life. They are not necessarily what we see on the news show, or hear from the radio, or read about in the newspaper, but they are what we know of our own personal lives. On the other hand, they are not moods, they are not thoughts, they are not plans, they are not our character, they are not our essence, nor our spirit. But they are related to all of these and other aspects of our nature as human beings. And of course, animals experience events just as humans do. Events are a universal and key ingredient in the lives of all living things.

In sum: For this particular event property of being discrete, the question you would ask yourself is, "Is this just a single event standing by itself, or does it involve and connect with other events?"

Events vary in magnitude. Some events that we experience are common and, relatively small in their impact on us. Choosing what breakfast cereal, what to wear, and what kind of TV show to watch are examples of such events. They are often easily resolved and then forgotten, while others may stick with us in our memory. But we also occasionally experience events much larger in their scope, although these are less frequent than small events. When these high impact major life events occur, they engage much more of our time and effort, and they can have a life-changing impact on us. Some are desirable like getting married or having a child, while others, oppositely valenced, are undesirable, such as having a car accident or experiencing the trauma of a battle injury. In the Introduction, I presented the story of Jeff Lewis, a Mesa, Arizona high school teacher, who was seriously injured by an accidental gunshot, clearly a "major life event." But the story only began there: He bounced back, later enjoying his new life as a multiple amputee, playing golf and dancing. Some people can display remarkable resilience in the face of a major negative event, while others retreat under the pressure. To explain these differences, research has compared the effects of small daily events and major life events, with surprising results which I will present.

In sum: For this particular event property of event magnitude, the question you would ask yourself is, "Is this a small daily event that I can easily handle, or is it major and going to require a lot of my resources to handle?"

Events vary in their chronicity (recurrence). Thinking of events as having a discrete beginning helps you regard them as distinct occurrences, but how they end, if they do, is an important additional distinction. Many events do not have a sharp, distinct ending such as a growing illness, a recurring infection from an injury, or a flare-up of a chronic illness like arthritis or experiencing chronic PTSD. On the positive side, a happy marriage infuses our life every day, while birthdays have a dependable recurrence once every year. This property of chronicity has an effective continuing influence on our ability to anticipate and prepare for each occurrence and this in turn helps us maintain our resilience and outlook on life. Sudden and unexpected event occurrences put stress on our coping capacity, while expected ones motivate us with anticipation and preparation, thereby strengthening our resilience when they occur.

In sum: For this particular event property of event chronicity, the question you would ask yourself is, "Is this a one-time event that I won't experience again, or is it going to occur again (and perhaps again)?"

Events vary in their emotional valence. Some events are desirable, others are undesirable. As I said in my opening comments at the beginning of this chapter, we seek things we want in our life and we seek to avoid things we do not want in our life. The research traditions studying events which I will present throughout this book uses the language of "desirable events" or "positive events" and "undesirable events" or "negative events" to investigate the relationships between the emotional feelings which are linked with the events in our lives. In turn, numerous studies show that they are linked with our physical and mental well-being. And of course some events are relatively neutral in their emotional feelings. Although they may not particularly stand out in our lives, research shows that experiencing them can have positive consequences for us under certain circumstances. Sometimes the effects of these events are counterintuitive: Some desirable events have been shown to cause negative consequences for us, while some negative events can have positive effects on our well-being if we approach them in a healthy, resilient manner. This book is all about what I mean by "dealing in a healthy resilient manner." It is complex, but it is doable once you see the underlying principles of how your life's events relate to your well-being.

In sum: For this event property of event valence, the question you would ask yourself is, "Is this a desirable event to be pursued, or an undesirable event to be avoided?"

Events vary in their causation. Sometimes you yourself will make an event occur, such as going to work or talking to a friend or brushing your teeth or going jogging. But other events arise because of the actions of other people or the world, and you play no causal role in making them occur. Research shows that the factor of causing an event to occur or, on the other hand, passively experiencing an event is the key consideration in assessing their role in our well-being. The social psychologist Richard DeCharms calls these conditions, "origin" and "pawn."

To be an origin of an event's causation is a very different type of psychological experience than to be a "pawn" of having the event "happen" to you. This book is aimed at helping you understand this critical distinction, and it is the key to the entire approach I am presenting in this book.

In sum: For this particular event property of event causation, the question you would ask yourself is, "Is this an event that I made occur, or is it an event caused by some force outside of my personal causation?"

A Realistic Understanding of Events in Our Lives

The evidence we have about events is based on scientific research. That means, in practice, that researchers have taken an "all else held constant" approach in their studies of events. To do that, they try to focus on one single event, isolated as much as possible from other events, and study its properties and the effects is has on people. For example, take "winning a lottery." That is a distinct, one-time occurrence, and we now know a lot about the effects such an experience has on people (see my discussion of this research in Chapter 5). But we know that all of us have many things going on in our lives all the time; at any given moment, in addition to winning the lottery, we are dealing with a set of immediately-present experiences, other short-term and longer-term goals we are expecting to occur, and there are other people with all of the events of their lives overlapping with our own lives and our own events. This is all quite complicated. Any single statement we make about a given event's effects on us has to be qualified by all of the other events which could themselves be a topic of study. So I want to declare here what I just said, that everything we know is true but "with all else held constant." But I also know that once you get the principles and main themes of what research has shown us, you will have a strong sense of how you can gain personal mastery over the events of your life no matter how complicated and confusing it may seem at times. You will develop a personal mastery template or map showing how you can guide your life through the complexities of your daily living.

Experiencing Events Can be Improved by Therapeutic Interventions

It turns out that understanding these event properties gives researchers and therapists powerful techniques for helping people improve their capacities for enhancing their event experiences. A body of psychological research has tested a wide variety of experimental treatments for enhancing our personal control over the events of our lives. These studies have shown that event-based treatments can be successful at enhancing participants' physical and mental health. The techniques are standardized and adaptable to the individual, and you can adopt some version of this general approach into your own lifestyle.

After I review some of the major therapeutic interventions which have been developed to test models of personal causation, in Chapter 9 I will describe an intervention which I conducted with my colleagues Alex Zautra and Mary Davis. It was based directly on the event properties I discuss in this and following chapters. It presents you with specific ways in which you can develop greater resilience in your life by being both an origin and a pawn, depending on the state of the world as you experience it.

Empowerment: Matching the Internal with the External

I asked earlier in this chapter, "Control Over What?" What is to be the aim of any empowerment treatment? The research literature has a clear answer to these questions. Paying more attention both to the inner mental world of a person plus putting a stronger focus on the external events in that person's life greatly expands our understanding of the value of the concept of empowerment. At first pass, the term would seem to imply strengthening a person's inner resources, skills, capacities, and resilience motivations. But all organisms live in an environment, a surrounding envelope of entities and events with their own existence independent of the person. In this external world are a myriad of experiences potentially supporting or harming our individual drives for personal empowerment. Only a model of empowerment which incorporates both your inner capacities and the external occurrences which you experience can provide a comprehensive understanding of how it is that you can take control over your life's events and enhance your own well-being. This book provides an inclusive coverage of *both* realms of factors and a model experiment showing how they can be integrated into a more effective lifestyle. Let us now begin the journey! Let us take our Jeff Lewis story as our guide.

Chapter 2

Mastery Regarded as a Character Trait

Jeff Lewis's story is so amazing that your first thought is one of admiration for his fortitude. But his story is so unusual that it seems that there must be something beyond just fortitude, but something basically fundamental about him as a person, his character, that led him to succeed in the face of such obstacles. After all, he did reach down deep and take control over his own life, handicap and all, and conquered what might sweep away many of us.

One common way that people account for his resilience is to say that "he's that kind of person." The implication of this kind of explanation is that the cause of his reactions to his stressful experience lay inside him, in his personality, in his traits and characteristic habits of thoughts and beliefs. In this line of reasoning, we would say that he has a high sense of *trait personal control*, or *trait personal mastery*. His resilience must be due to some inner, stable, enduring pattern of causation that would generalize across many different aspects of his life, including his accident. A similar line of reasoning would be used to explain the behavior of, for instance, optimists or pessimists, or high intelligence or low intelligence people, or people who are highly sociable or loners. There is a myriad of descriptions we have to explain stable, enduring patterns of people's behavior that is consistent across times and situations. Indeed, such line of reasoning is nearly universal and familiar in our everyday interactions with our family, friends, and of course our perceptions of public figures even if we do not know them personally.

In that spirit of trait-based explanations of behavior, I am devoting the first part of this chapter to reviewing the body of research on trait personal mastery. Later in the chapter I will devote discussion to an event-based approach to our personal mastery beliefs and the actual personal control we have, or do not have, over the events of our lives. Both the trait approach and the event-control approach play a key role in our mental and physical health. But the topic of control and mastery beliefs as rooted in stable personality processes is a foundation of a good deal of psychological research and clinical practice, and it is the first topic to be presented in this chapter.

This kind of reasoning about the internal causes of behavior, at least in our modern times, goes all the way back to the early days of Sigmund Freud where the causes of our behavior were assumed to be located in our unconscious. More modern thinking has abandoned such fatalistic language but nevertheless continues his search for more enduring and stable characteristics. That quest was taken up in social and personality psychology research. One of the most influential waves of that research tradition was focused specifically on a person's control over the events in his or her life. This classic research revolved around what came to be called the "locus of control." As you can tell from the name, the emphasis of this line of reasoning sought to investigate the location (locus) of a person's perceptions of their own ability to achieve goals of significance to them. In this view, people have stable inner dispositions that allow them to determine their own courses of actions across time and situations and, especially, environments. I will present some sample personality test items assessing such beliefs shortly. People who score high on this trait are called "internals" because they perceive the causal source of their actions to be inside of them, as a stable disposition in their personality makeup. Of course not everyone is an "internal." It is a continuum and some people are more tempered or moderate in their beliefs. But some people have very little of this trait. By tradition they are called "externals," because they believe that events in their lives are caused not by themselves, but by forces outside of themselves, in their physical environment, by other people and, often, by luck and chance (fate).

These categories are not necessarily hard and fast, but they do give you an idea of the general orientations that people come to believe about themselves and how they believe that they can or cannot control the events in their life. These beliefs are subtle and they are not something that we usually think about on a daily basis. But when something gets out of your control and you cannot control the outcome, then you really get a sense of how critical this kind of belief actually is to your well-being. I will soon discuss a good deal of evidence which supports exactly that point.

The initial studies on the concept of locus of control ignited a firestorm of research, leading to over 2,000 publications in the past 50 years! It is surely one of the most-researched concepts ever studied in the social sciences. After all these decades, the research findings are highly consistent, at least in Western cultures, in showing that control has major positive effects on mental and physical health.

The simplest way to find out a person's sense of mastery or control is to ask them. Of course, there are highly technical ways to do that. That is basically what psychologists who specialize in the science of *psychometrics* do. In this branch of the social sciences, particularly psychology, researchers and clinical practitioners traditionally employ so-called "self-report" pencil-and-paper questionnaire items which tap into internal and external control beliefs. They then employ sophisticated statistical techniques to develop a quantitative scoring scale which assesses some state or condition of the person that can be standardized and used to establish reliable norms for the population of interest.

The IQ test is the supreme example of refined psychometrics that give us a way to use people's verbal responses to standard questions with which we can then array their responses from low (little or none of the trait or characteristic) on up to "very high" of that trait. When we say that someone "has" a high IQ, that is easily translated into scale scores, let's say, 125 or higher. It is a statistical statement, actually, but it has a lot of personal, social and cultural meanings that give us a good idea of how that person can perform in a wide range of situations.

That is what psychologists have done for measuring people's control beliefs. Ellen Skinner[1] has surveyed this extensive body of research and has shown that there are many variations on this theme; she has described research using 100 different scales to measure personal control! There are three general orientations that these approaches take to control: (1) Believing that you do or do not possess the means to achieve your goals, represented by the self-efficacy and "human agency" model of Albert Bandura[2,3] (2) believing that the means you possess will or will not achieve a goal, the "contingency judgment" model of John Weisz and Deborah Stipek,[4] and the "explanatory style" model of Lynn Abramson, Martin Seligman and John Teasdale,[5] and (3) believing that you can directly control your outcomes, the "perceived control" model of Skinner herself.[6] These distinctions are helpful for understanding the range of applicability of control concepts and they are important to technical researchers, but for my purposes I will use the blanket terms of either "personal control" or "personal mastery" without drawing such fine distinctions in my discussion.

Next, I am going to present some sample items from some of the more popular scales to give you an idea of how psychologists have come to think of this general dimension of personality. I will not deal in any great detail with the specific differences among the various scales, although there are key facets that will be important to discuss later on. Right now, here is a brief description of some of the more popular "LOC" scales.

Generalized Beliefs in One's Personal Control

Julian Rotter[7] developed the most influential measurement scale specifically designed to assess personal control beliefs. Thinking that it would be most clearly related to how a person believed in their ability (or lack of it) to obtain good outcomes in their lives, he constructed a set of paired choices in which the person is to pick the one that most accurately represented their own personal feelings. Here are several of the paired choices. You might read them over and think about how you would pick one of each pair as most closely representing what you think about yourself and your life.

1a. *In my case getting what I want has little or nothing to do with luck.*

1b. *Many times we must just as well decide what to do by flipping a coin.*

2a. *As far as world affairs are concerned, most of us are the victims of forces we can neither understand nor control.*

2b. *By taking an active part in political and social affairs, the people can control world events.*

3a. *I have often found that what is going to happen will happen.*

3b. *Trusting in fate has never turned out as well for me as making a decision to take a definite course of action.*

4a. *Many times I feel that I have little influence over the things that happen to me.*

4b. *It is impossible for me to believe that chance or luck play an import role in my life.*

As you can tell from reading over these examples, there are two ways in which control is being assessed in each of these paired choices: One is to state directly that you the person (or people in general) can control the events of their lives; the other choice in the pair suggests that you or people in general do not have control. By tradition in the research literature, the first grouping of items is thought of as assessing internal control, and the second deals with external control. Now that you have read how the scale is constructed, and how your answers fit those items, you might be able to see which end or the middle of the scale best matches your thoughts about how you get along in life. Keep in mind, though, that Rotter distinctly thought of his scale as assessing generalized control beliefs, so he is dealing with an overall tendency across all items rather than any specific instances that might come to your mind as you read the items.

As I said at the end of Chapter 1, research necessarily deals with average tendencies. We are dealing here with general patterns and trends of responses, not necessarily specific item-by-item interpretations and qualifications that might lead to endless debate in your own mind about how well an item fits specific instances that you might recall. The scale is intended to give you a general picture of your beliefs about how your world "works," to use the language of personal causation. Once again, let me point out that this language may be unfamiliar to you. We are not used to thinking of our self in the terms of generalized beliefs like this. But the proof comes in how this line of reasoning makes sense to us as we see the consequences of research using it.

Another popular scale is that of Leonard Pearlin and Carmi Schooler[8] which they labeled "The Personal Mastery Scale." It contains [7] items which the person is to state how often they have been feeling that way in the past month (from "Not at all" to "Very much"):

1. *There is really no way I can solve some of the problems I have.*
2. *Sometimes I feel that I'm being pushed around in life.*
3. *I have little control over the things that happen to me.*
4. *I can do just about anything I really set my mind to.*
5. *I often feel helpless in dealing with the problems of life.*

6. *What happens to me in the future mostly depends on me.*
7. *There is little I can do to change many of the important things in my life.*

As you can see, items 4 and 6 indicate that the person has a high degree of belief in their mastery over their life events, whereas the other items indicate just the opposite, that the person believes that they have little or no control over the events of their life. How would you respond to these items? Again, keep in mind that these items are to be regarded as tapping into your general beliefs rather than any specific instances of occurrences in your life.

Now that you have seen the two major foundational approaches to your control beliefs, I want to set down a simple ground rule for how I have handled the many different terms and concepts in the vast research literature on personal causation. You will note that I have already used several different terms: "locus of control," "personal control" and "personal mastery". They can be interpreted to mean slightly different concepts, and each term has been employed many times by many investigators in studies of many outcomes. In the interest of reviewing for you the vast range of studies on these topics, I will not necessarily mean one particular scale to the exclusion of the other as I present the findings of these studies. For my purpose, it is sufficient to use one term or another at any given point in the discussion. The differences in these concepts are much less interesting than the similarities, and I will use the terms interchangeably from here on out.

Beliefs for Specific Classes of Personal Control

Many researchers and clinical practitioners immediately saw the value in adapting the personal mastery/control perspective for understanding and enhancing people's well-being. With these scales as a foundational approach, a number of investigators sought to develop tests for applying assessment of control beliefs to specific domains of people's lives. A few of the many tests that were developed for research and clinical applications were such topics as control over your academic achievement, control over your physical health, including obesity, marital satisfaction, achievement in sports, and for controlling one's economic status, even politics. One entire area of research involved developing and testing scales that are appropriate for children. There are too many specific applications for me to discuss them all, but some representative ones will give you an idea of how powerful and how useful this way of thinking can be.

One of the better-researched of these specific types of control tests is the Health Locus of Control Scale by Kenneth Wallston and his colleagues.[9] Here are some examples from subscales of their test.

1. *If I get sick, it is my own behavior which determines how soon I get well again.*
2. *When I get sick I am to blame.*
3. *Health professionals control my health.*
4. *My family has a lot to do with my becoming sick or staying healthy.*
5. *No matter what I do, if I am going to get sick, I will get sick.*

May Keyson and Lou Janda[10] worked extensively with alcoholics and developed a scale to measure the person's sense of control over their drinking. They used the forced choice technique that Julian Rotter used in his original scale where people have to make a choice between one of two opposite choices which best represent their thinking and feeling on the particular issue. Here are a few examples of their paired-choice items.

1a. *Successfully licking alcoholism is a matter of hard work, luck has little or nothing to do with it.*

1b. *Staying sober depends mainly on things going right for you.*

2a. *I feel powerless to prevent myself from drinking when I am anxious or unhappy.*

2b. *If I really wanted to, I could stop drinking.*

3a. *I have control over my drinking behavior.*

3b. *I feel completely helpless when it comes to resisting a drink.*

4a. *Drink isn't necessary in order to solve my problems.*

4b. *I just cannot handle my problems unless I take a drink first.*

As you can tell, assessing a person's beliefs in their capacity for controlling their lives are pretty straightforward. The items are immediately clear in their intent, and people seem to have a good understanding of their own beliefs to be able to give consistent and reliable answers. Those are the hallmarks of good assessment instruments.

What about the Mental and Physical Health of High vs. Low Control People?

Researchers and therapists immediately saw the power of this approach to reveal complex but subtle facets of the adjustment and well-being of samples of people who score high or low on the particular assessment instrument. One of the major areas of investigation involved physical health, and here the studies have generated impressively consistent results. Surveys by some of the leading researchers in the field Bonnie Strickland,[11,12] Margaret Lachman[13] and Barbara and Kenneth Wallston,[14] all reveal that high internal people are more motivated to protect and enhance their physical health, they guard against accidents more than externals, and they engage in better precautionary activities such as greater amounts of exercise. Their high levels of beliefs in their own personal control protect them against developing PTSD symptoms.[15] Having strong beliefs in one's effectiveness leads to a better ability to distinguish between safe and risky situations.[16] They also rate their own health better than externals rate theirs and they report having fewer limitations in their functioning in daily activities.[11] More physiologically, they are less likely to have heart attacks and they have better responses to medical treatment.[18] Judith Rodin and Christine Timko[19] reported that health surveys on samples of medical patients indicated that highly internal people know more about their medical condition and are more willing than externals to attend patient education classes.

In the realm of addiction research, the personal control approach again has proven helpful. In a sample of smokers trying to quit smoking, internals were more successful than externals in reducing their cigarette consumptions and they were better at maintaining their reduction. In alcohol addiction studies, Stanley Butts and John Chotlos[20] found that a sample of males in an alcohol treatment program scored more in the external direction compared to a carefully matched sample of nonalcoholics. Dennis Donovan and Michael O'Leary[21] reported that external alcoholics tend to be more depressed than internal alcoholics. Even among nonalcoholics who do drink occasionally, the more external people tend to drink more, showing some motivation to reduce negative feelings in their lives.

Research on mental health assessments show similar effects of high internal control beliefs. A summary of a number of studies on personal control and depression, a meta-analysis by Victor Benassi, Paul Sweeney and Charles Dufour,[22] found that higher levels of external locus of control beliefs were related to greater depression. A very recent summary of studies in 18 cultural regions around the world, with a total of 33,224 adults reported that external control beliefs were significantly related to high depression and, independently, high feelings of anxiety.[23] The relationship between external locus of control and anxiety in college students as a separate sample has been found in a study by Irwin Sandler and Brian Lakey,[24] so the connection appears to be a strong one.

A nationwide study of middle-aged adults showed that more internal beliefs were associated with greater life satisfaction. High internality people were more optimistic in their approach to adulthood, and they expected things to stay that way or even improve. Higher internality people have a greater capacity for responding to stresses such as economic downturns,[25] they are less stressed by losing a job,[26] and they are more capable of handling the burdens of caregiving.[27] A large-scale national survey of German citizens covering 25 years of assessment showed that those residents who scored higher in personal beliefs lived significantly longer than those who scored lower.[28] In terms of physical health, people without physical illnesses report lower levels of depressive symptoms, but those who report some degree of illness report lower levels of depression when they are feeling higher levels of mastery.[29]

Cognitive processes, in the sense of information processing, also show a difference between internals and externals. A higher sense of personal control relates to a number of different types of cognitive performances and activities. For instance, several studies have shown that internals prefer games of skill over games of chance, whereas externals prefer to engage in chance activities.[30,31] Internals tend to be more attentive and alert and to process information more effectively for problem solutions.[32] In situations where there is social pressure to conform to a group standard, externals are more likely to conform than internals, who are more independent.[33] Internals are more likely to be involved in political activism.[7] In work settings, employees who score higher on internality hold higher-level managerial positions; conversely, professionals who are more highly trained than other employees score higher on internality than workers who have nonsupervisory positions and less skill.[34] High internals tend to rate their job satisfaction higher and they rated higher in actual job performance.[35]

But What about Control in the Environment?

I have presented these results concerning the characteristics of personal control as if the person lived in a vacuum. But researchers who have focused on personal mastery and control beliefs are quite aware of the power of the environment. No matter how much a person may be an internal or an external, in the sense of having a particular type of personality or trait as an enduring disposition, nevertheless our picture would not be complete unless we acknowledge that the environment itself has controlling properties.

This concept is so important for our purposes that it needs deeper consideration. Economists speak of the "financial environment," architects speak of the "built environment," and public policy experts of the "political environment." These different approaches to the concept of "environment" all have as a common model consideration of the "surround" of their topic of particular interest. They are all referring to the set of elements which create the space within which their topic operates and functions. Psychologists also are concerned with understanding the elements surrounding the behavior of people. In personal mastery and control research, "the environment" is considered to be *that space which contains all of the events and occurrences to which the person responds.* This conceptualization makes possible quantitative and qualitative research on discrete, observable, and measureable events in the person's living space.

In research on personal control, the focus is shifted from strictly inside the person to the daily occurrences that fill our day and major events. This is the main feature of the event-based approach I introduced in Chapter 1. But the term also refers to *situations or conditions* of the person's existence.

An environment of low controlling conditions would be a condition of a high degree of free choice for the person, with few external constraints. For example, imagine going on a shopping trip or going to a bookstore. One can browse the stores or the books and buy or not buy, depending almost entirely on one's own personal choices and decisions; the situation does not force you to do anything. But a "high controlling environment" would be a very different environment for our sense of mastery. For instance, imagine being in a prison. You have little freedom of choice there; the control resides in the system of rules and regulations, not in free choice by the person. Nursing homes keep control over their residents. Schools keep control over their students in the classroom. The military deliberately restricts freedom of recruits until their recruits' training is completed at which time it is expected that discipline will be ingrained and control moved "inside" the person. Even then, though, there is a chain of command and those persons lower in the chain, no matter how they would score on a scale of internal-external control, are expected to "follow orders."

So what would happen if a person high in personal control were to be put in a highly controlling environment? How would a person who believes in external control respond in an unstructured environment offering few restraints and control? The questions derive from what is called the "Person by Environment" (PXE) research tradition or, alternatively, "Person by Environment fit" or "congruence" research. The main question here is to determine the effects of the match or congruence between the person's trait of personal control, high or low, and the degree of control pressures ongoing or relatively absent in a particular environment. To give you a picture of this type of approach I will review briefly some relevant PXE areas of research and clinical practice.

The Environment of the Therapy Setting

Clinical psychologists have been interested in the internal-external sense of control in their patients and the type of therapy that would be most effective for their patients. The types of therapies that clinicians employ to help their clients vary from highly structured and carefully controlled by the therapist to more open and unstructured, allowing the clients more freedom in their treatment. One study tested for the effectiveness of these two types of therapies for internal *vs.* external participants who had responded to locus of control scales prior to beginning their therapies.[36] Significant interaction effects were found. The internal participants in the structured sessions later became less cooperative and more avoiding, whereas the external participants showed more benefits from the structured treatment approach. This supports the personal control approach by suggesting that more internal participants will do better in more unstructured settings which allow them more freedom of choice and action.

The Environment of the Business Setting

Business settings are a good environment to study PXE effects. Some businesses allow employees high degrees of participation whereas others restrict participation. These situations should have different effects on employees depending on their trait personal control. Peter Brownell[37] recruited College of Business students to participate in a business game simulation in which they were to construct a budget plan for a product. Control was created when the participants were told that their own decision would carry great weight in the final decision accepted by top management, *versus* another group was told that their decision would carry little weight in top management's decision. Participants' scores on the Rotter Internal-External control scale were assessed. In agreement with what theory would predict, the high internal control participants performed better and enjoyed participating more than low control participants in the high personal influence condition. The same was true of the high external participants in the low-participation condition; they performed better and had greater enjoyment. Those results show that congruence of person and situation (PXE) leads to better performance and satisfaction, whereas incongruence of person and situation leads to poorer performance and satisfaction. This dual approach to both personal control and environment control is a very powerful way to understand our daily experiences and how they relate to our well-being.

Control Over Positive and Negative Events

Now let me turn to how this approach links up with the events of our daily experiences. Probing the nature of control in terms of achieving control over positive events and avoiding negative ones, Fred Bryant[38] developed questionnaire items to assess each class of valence events separately, and then tested for Rotter I-E differences in endorsing those beliefs. To assess control over positive events, he developed the "Obtaining" scale with such items as:

In general, how much control do you feel that you personally have over whether or not good things happen to you?

With respect to good thing that have occurred in your life, to what extent do you think that you have typically been responsible for their occurrence?

To assess beliefs in the ability to avoid negative events, he developed the "Avoiding" scale. Here are some representative items from that scale:

In general, how much control do you feel that you personally have over whether or not bad things happen to you?

In general, how likely or unlikely do you think it is that bad things will happen to you?

In a study of 47 college students, he found that those who rated higher in internality as a personality trait scored higher on the Obtaining scale (for positive events) and also scored lower on the Avoiding scale (for negative events). Combining scores for the I-E scale, his data also showed that people who scored higher on the Obtaining scale scored higher in other measures of positive emotions, and those who scored higher on the Avoiding scale scored higher on measures of psychological distress. So there is consistent evidence that internal-external control beliefs are related to believing in one's ability to make desirable events occur in one's life and to block undesirable events from occurring. But perceived control is, in general, two-pronged: Believing that one can create desirable events and prevent undesirable events is *both* related to measures of mental health and well-being (but of course in opposite directions).

The Environment of the Social Network

Our social environment can be interpreted from an event causation perspective. "Social situations" can come from other people as well as therapy sessions or organizational structures. People in our social environment can be thought of as providing social events for us that support our drives for control or they can be providing situations which encourage us to let them control our own personal events; the effect of this is to make us dependent and reliant on them. This could be called "social control" as a specific type of control we experience and it pervades our daily living, even though we may not be aware of it as such.

As an example of when people either "control" us by either encouraging us to "do it your way" *vs.* "here, do it my way," you can see how independence from or dependence on them is the underlying message they are giving us. A classic example, and in fact one which guided my own research, is physical health. When people become ill, there is a natural tendency for other people to want to help them, to provide for their needs, do things for them, and in general to "take care" of them during their illness. Of course, those same "controlling" behaviors might not be appropriate for a healthy person, one whose sense of personal mastery is not under stress due to physical illness: To encourage *dependence* rather than *independence* might be unwelcome. But the perspective I am using here follows the same logic: There might be a PXE interaction, in which high internal control people would respond well to their social relationships which encourage them to be independent, while external control people would respond well if their social environment encouraged dependence.

Be aware, of course, that what I just said has a distinctly "Western" bias to it: Oriental people may not value rugged individualism and personal independence to the extent that Western culture people do. This is a big topic of concern in anthropology, sociology, and social psychology, but I want instead to focus on interpersonal control processes here.

So with the collaboration of my clinician/researcher colleagues Alex Zautra and Mary Davis, I began a series of studies on personal control, physical illness, and social situations of internal control (encouraging independence) and external social control (encouraging dependence). Physical illness often is debilitating and leaves us with activity limitations which constrain our freedom of action. Although very common, an illness can leave us with conditions which restrict our freedom of action representing real threats to our beliefs in our personal control.

In our studies, all of our research participants were diagnosed by their physicians as having either rheumatoid arthritis or fibromyalgia, with both disorders characterized by widespread bodily pain, poor treatment possibilities and uncertain prognosis for improvement. This is a definite threat to personal control for many people, particularly as they age. Since these illnesses are heavily preponderant in females, all of our participants were female, although we also recruited their spouses to participate and give us reports on their controlling behavior toward their wives.

We assessed the patients' physical health and mental health to study the relations between their health outcomes and their spouses' controlling behaviors. In these studies, we were following a general PXE congruence model, and we carefully measured the personal control beliefs of the participants in our projects. However, to conduct a genuine PXE study, we went one step further and had the participants report on how much their *spouses* (in these projects, their major caregivers) had been encouraging independence or dependence. In some studies the participants themselves reported on the control characteristics of their spouses, but we also actually recruited the spouses themselves to report on their own behavior to their ill spouse, providing a very high degree of measurement validity to our models of social control.

The items we employed in these studies were very well developed by my graduate student Robert Grossman in his doctoral dissertation.[39] One set of items was designed to assess what we called "self-reliance encouragement" (SRE) scored in terms of how often the spouse had provided that support in the past month:

1. *Told her she should make her own decisions.*
2. *Suggested that she should work on her problems in her own way.*
3. *Told her that she can pretty much determine what will happen in her life.*
4. *Asked her to 'stand on her own feet,' emotionally.*
5. *Encourage her to be more self-reliant.*

Three items were designed to assess what we called, "other reliance encouragement" (ORE).

1. *Suggested that she be more reliant on others.*
2. *Encouraged her to feel that others know what's best for her.*
3. *Suggested that she let others take more responsibility for solving her problems.*
4. *Suggested that others may be more capable of handling her problems than she is.*

Without going into detailed presentation of the complex data analyses these studies entailed, I can present the highlights of the more revealing of our findings.[40] In one study of a sample of patients recruited from a rheumatology practice the results showed that most of the significant influence of spousal SREORE occurred for externals. This was as we predicted, since people who believe that control is outside of themselves should be more sensitive to control attempts coming from other people. When their husbands were encouraging independence (SRE), those patients who were older and in poorer physical health responded with feelings of greater depression, anxiety, and other facets of poorer mental health; self-reliance encouragement did not fit well with their personality disposition, a PXE interpretation. But those patients whose husbands had been encouraging higher levels of self-reliance (SRE) reported better mental health if they were younger in age and in relatively better health.

Note that all of the effects were happening in the more external participants; those who had more internal beliefs were relatively unaffected by their husbands' social control efforts. So while as Westerners we might think that dependence encouragement would not have a positive effect on someone, these data show that it has positive benefits for people who do not think that they have high levels of personal control in their lives (they are externals), when they are older and when they are in poorer health.

These results suggested that externality, per se, gives a slant toward greater sensitivity to the behavior of other people. In a second study[41] we wanted to know more about dependence encouragement. We assessed it (ORE) with an expanded scale with more questions (*e.g., "Answered question for her that medical staff asked her"* and, *"Discouraged friends and family from visiting when she was not feeling well."*) Again we asked the husbands to report on their own behavior toward their wives. We again found that ORE effects were significant for the external patients but not for the internals. The data showed that higher levels of dependence encouragement tended to lower the feelings of psychological distress in external patients who had more recently experienced physical downturns from their illness. But the longer they had been diagnosed with their illness, and presumably better adjusted to its stresses, then higher ORE led to greater distress; being encouraged to be reliant on others had negative consequences for them.

Overall, encouraging medical patients to be dependent on others leads to improved mental health if they had more recently experienced symptoms and were older, but to poorer mental health if they were relatively healthier and younger. Despite what one might initially think, overprotectiveness on the part of a spouse can be helpful for rheumatoid arthritis patients who have recently had a health downtown or are older in age.

Other researchers have found results similar to ours, so they have been tested in other samples and found to be reliable. Vicki Helgeson[42] studied cardiac patients and spousal caregiving and found that, at the initial onset, protectiveness by the spouse has positive benefits, but when it goes on later in the recovery period, it tends to have negative effects. These studies show that influential social effects are found when we account for the patients' beliefs in their own high (or low) levels of personal control.

Caregivers have a natural tendency to want to help, to do something for someone suffering physical problems. While noble in intent, and while this mode of caregiving sometimes does have overall positive effects, these studies show that "help" is not always helpful. "Helping" is tricky, and as I said in Chapter 1, that trickiness is complex and often subtle in how it can work for the best benefit of the patient. One size definitely does not fit all in this complicated world of physical illness and social events.

Two Classes of Personal Control

Caution in interpreting and applying any research is always advisable, a point that Dean Shapiro, Carolyn Schwartz, and John Astin demonstrated in their extensive review of the research and clinical literature.[43] One can believe too strongly in one's ability to control events; as you will see in later chapters, many of the events of our lives simply are not amenable to our attempts to control them. On the other hand, not believing that you can assert some form of control over some events in your life can lead to poor utilization of one's real strength. From any perspective, life is a complex balancing act of many aspects of our selves and of our environment. Estimating the effectiveness of one's control attempts has to be judged in light of the nature of the situation itself, the main thrust of any interactional approach.

At the same time, there is another angle on PXE interactional models. Treating personal control as an enduring trait only captures a part of the richness of the concept. Sometimes most of us at times think that we can control things and at other times we think we cannot, and these feelings are not rigid and inflexible; they can change, depending on the situation and on our other physical and mental conditions. In spite of its long historical development and its impressive success in accounting for a wide range of outcomes, nevertheless personal control need not be thought solely of as a stable, unchangeable aspect of the person's personality. The PXE tradition thus opens up a wider range of ways to think about control: Control as a specific possibility, or not, in a specific environment.

This line of reasoning led Fred Rothbaum, John Weisz, and Samuel Snyder to develop one of the most important shifts in scientific thinking about personal control. In what has become a classic rethinking of the concept, they entitled their publication, "Changing the World and Changing the Self: A Two-Process Model of Perceived Control,"[44] indicating that the classical meaning of the term needs to be expanded to uncontrollable situations where, in fact, the individual has a range of alternative responses that in and of themselves represent a different form of control. As you can see from their title, they expand the concept from the basic meaning of "bringing the world into line with our wishes" but situations in which we deliberately give up this *primary* form of control and change over into a wide range of other control techniques. In their classic phrase, you can change your world or you can change your self (literally, your "self'"). You have many ways to bring yourself into line with the world. This is a form of deliberate accommodation, in the sense of adjusting yourself to events, going with the situation as it presents itself to us, and thus retaining your self-integrity. The famous 12-step program of Alcoholics Anonymous adopted the Niebuhr Serenity Prayer. By having AA participants personally endorse the organization's statement that they one can no longer control their own drinking; that statement and adopting that statement as one's own belief, then the AA member had made a firm assertion of personal control by yielding to an external, superior force, the compulsion to drink. This is a necessary first step in restoring and building one's sense of what we now would call primary control. This distinction directs personal control over events and accommodating yourself to an unchangeable world is a major advancement in psychological science and therapeutic practice, and I return to it again at the end of Chapter 9.

Eastern philosophies are replete with similar concepts. Giving oneself over to the world in order to gain transcendence and meaning in life shows the value of having a flexible use of control concepts. Beth Morling and Sharrilyn Evered[45] and Ellen Skinner[46] have explored the various facets of these other types of control, and they reject the idea that these alternative forms of adjustment are somehow secondary to anything. You can choose to be passive, to go with the flow and have no thoughts of trying to control your environment. After all, listening to music is a rewarding and enriching experience in which you completely give over your self to your environment. Donald Hodges[47] has recently summarized a large body of research showing the undeniably positive effects of listening to music on our mental health and well-being. One does not have to be a performer (controlling an instrument) to gain great benefits of "going with the flow."

So there clearly are benefits to accommodating yourself to uncontrollable external events. But although resignation and passivity sometimes seem easy ways to accommodate, if carried too far they can lead to a serious withdrawal from important daily events, and as I will show in Chapter 5, we can become consumed with a sense of helplessness and depression. These are not necessary outcomes of dealing with uncontrollable events, but they are potential outcomes if we do not actively choose accommodation and acceptance as our healthy ways of adapting to unchangeable events. We can think of control as changing your thoughts, your motivations, your choices, *etc.* if your attempts at direct control are not successful. Jurgen Brandstetter and Klaus Rothermund[48] discussed the differences in these two types of PXE situations. Personal control over achieving your goals is more likely to be successful when, (1) the events are controllable, (2) you have the actions and resources available to sustain your goal pursuit, and your goals are high priority. But when those conditions are not met, then you are more likely to be successful when (1) the events are not controllable, (2) your actions and resources are not as available as needed, and (3) you have alternative goals that can be satisfying as substitutes.

However we choose to think of it, these approaches to the alternative ways we have available to us as we deal with out of control events has given us ways to think of how we can match our own motivations and behaviors with the realities of the world in which we find ourselves. As you know by now, we define that world as one resulting from our own personal causation, or as one resulting from forces outside of us. Coming to incorporate that two-category picture of PXE fit processes is a much richer and more realistic way of thinking about how we retain a sense of mastery in, basically, any environment. In order to make clearer all of the various components that go into our successful dealing with events under our control and those arising outside of us, I have developed a schematic diagram or picture of how these components interrelate. In order to see all of the various parts, the next 5 chapters are devoted to reviewing research and theory on desirable and undesirable events and how we deal with them, successfully or not. The diagram is presented in Chapter 8.

A Definition of Personal Control

So, in sum, there is a fundamental, basic distinction that will be important to your thinking throughout this book. It is a distinction that will become a part of your template of personal control that you adopt as you move forward in your life from this point on. That distinction is between your control over the events in your life and your lack of it, controllable events and uncontrollable events. But there is an important qualification to that distinction. If you confront uncontrollable events or situations, then we know that you can switch to accommodation, adjustment, and acceptance and many other forms of changing your self. So when the Serenity Prayer which speaks of "the courage to change the things I can," Niebuhr probably was not thinking of the many distinctions researchers have now shown to be very important as we confront changing events in our lives.

The distinction between "courage to change things" can now be thought of as the choice we have to attempt to change. "Courage" may be more acceptable if we think of it as flexibility in our choices and actions, based on a fundamental understanding of the nature of events and their properties which I discussed earlier in Chapter 1. The template for your personal mastery I am helping you to develop will be your fallback, your default option, when life gets confusing and you are faced with a set of events than you can comfortably handle at that moment. It can help you see ways to achieve desirable events and avoid undesirable events by finding their controllability, under your control or not. And it can help you to understand the life of other people as they pursue the same goals.

Sometimes common sense and cultural truisms can become disconnected from the realities of life and become misleading, if not actually harmful. One particularly well-known instance which I think deserves reconsideration in the light of personal mastery theory and research is the common cliché, "if at first you don't succeed, try and try again." No one can doubt the wisdom of perseverance and diligent pursuit of our goals. But that can become narrow-mindedness or fixation or, at the extreme, obsession. The event property of event causation should always be high in one's consciousness and the notion that our personal efforts will make an unchangeable event into a changeable one is a serious miscalculation. I will discuss the downside of that issue when I review research on, for instance, cancer patients and arthritis patients (in Chapter 4) who are facing a condition that will not change by "trying," while that same research shows that there are changeable components of such illnesses. Recovery is more effective when we focus our efforts on changing what is changeable, and sometimes it is better to put changing the self as the top priority in one's choices of how to live.

One more instance of cultural beliefs deserves a comment. You will recall the children's story of *The Little Engine That Could*. That case does in fact show the value of perseverance and high motivation to assert personal mastery over the environment, bringing the world into line with one's needs and desires. One has to conclude that the situation of going up the steep hill was in fact controllable, so high effort was rewarded with the end effect of "bringing the world under one's control." To extend our personal mastery template to this situation, I have to assume that the Little Engine was an "internal," as opposed to an external.

As I reviewed personality assessment instruments earlier in this chapter, thinking of personal control as a set of beliefs somehow lodged deep in the personality and trait structure has proved to be a productive way to think about a person's approach to life. Especially, that way of thinking tells us important pivot-points for understanding their adjustment and well-being. But that approach limits us to somewhat artificial groupings of people, such as those who are "highs" or "lows" on the trait of personal mastery. But everyone can be thought of as individuals, each of us as actively pursuing our own personal goals in life, not as just members of a class, as productive as that way of thinking has been. The important key is to find the linking between a person's quest for happiness in their life and the affordances in the environment in which they are acting. A broader approach to this approach to personal control would be useful for that type of thinking. One of the founders of the personal control tradition in research and clinical practice is Judith Rodin. I will cite some of her research later on. But her definition of this field I find to be inclusive and comprehensive enough to tap full range of the most important components of this approach. She defines it this way:

> Perceived control refers to the expectations of being able to participate in making decisions and engaging in actions in order to obtain desirable consequences and avoid unfavorable ones.[49]

Some Cautions and Broader Considerations

As you know, science tends to refine its procedures to get the sharpest picture of its topic, in this case personal mastery. So in reviewing the research on internal and external control, and I have described what we know of people who score as an "internal" or an "external" on some particular response scale. But when we apply that thinking to the real world, we run into some obvious pitfalls of that way of thinking. Life is of course not so simple. Although the findings are valid, they are only single findings and in no way can summarize all that a person is. We are more complicated than our single score on a questionnaire, no matter how compelling the various research studies may be. Fortunately, researchers have recognized this and have written extensively about how we can move from our single studies to a broader view of "real people in the real world." I want to review briefly what two major researchers in this area have written.

First, I have already cited the research of Bonnie Strickland earlier in this chapter. Her studies show the positive health benefits of internal control. But she also points out[12] that a person can believe too strongly in their own sense of control, that they can overestimate their control. Not everything in life is controllable, and to believe too strongly in one's control can be a mistake. She shows that in some cases exerting too much control can lead to coronary heart disease. The well-known Type A personality can show such effects. So we have to temper our discussion of this topic by acknowledging that a broader picture of the person in their environment is necessary.

Paul Wong and Catherine Sproule[50] have raised another issue with this way of thinking. Although our research talks about being an internal or an external (that is the way the data are computed in research studies), we have to think about people as being an internal *and* an external. We can answer both sets of questions in a survey and we can get a score on *both* variables. So any given person can be high or low or medium on the items assessing internality, and that person also can get a high, low, or medium score on items assessing externality. They want us to think of people as "bilocals," that is, we have two loci of causation sets of ideas and beliefs about our personal control. Wong and Sproule argue that it simply is not realistic to assume that if you are an internal you, therefore, automatically, will be low on external control beliefs. You can have all combinations of both scores, automatically. This is a very rich view of how we develop and maintain our beliefs about our personal control in life. This way of thinking opens up entire new vistas for conducting research studies, but I want to bring their valuable insights to the fore as you think about how these processes describe your own beliefs and your own personal lifestyle.

Getting a Picture of Events and How We Experience Them

So let us now start seeing how this kind of thinking has paid off in such a productive view of human health and well-being. We will start in the next chapter with a view to how the environment of the person fits with this set of beliefs about our personal mastery in our environment of events.

In the next chapter, I will review more of the research on both the person and the environment and their close connections.

Again I want to focus on the physical and mental well-being of people as they go about their daily lives. It will not surprise you to find out that control beliefs are, again, powerful determinants of how we respond to our world and the benefits, and the unpleasant costs, of how those beliefs operate for us.

Chapter 3

What Events Can Tell Us about Our Mastery

In the previous chapter I showed some of the many ways that we can think about mastery as if it were a trait or personal characteristic inside the person. But the concept is inclusive and it opens up many ways for us to think abut the environment in which the person carries on the activities of daily living. That is where my previous discussion of four major properties of events can become so useful in seeing how we negotiate the relationship between who we are and what kind of world of events fills our environment. In this chapter I want to delve much more deeply into the properties of events and what research has shown us about how those properties influence our well-being.

The accidental shooting of Jeff Lewis raises our sights to pay attention to the environment itself, independent of any person's personality traits, as important as these are. I think anyone judging the impact of his experience would regard it above all as *stressful*. Our personal mastery approach suggests a good deal about many of the important sources of our stress. When we go out into the environment surrounding that person, we will find there events which have positive or negative effects on that person's physical and mental well-being. The important question is, what have we learned about these properties of events that we can then use to get a better understanding of how they relate to our sense of personal mastery?

Given the great diversity of interests among researchers and therapists, event properties have been related to a wide range of outcome processes. Broadly speaking, investigators have wanted to study what might be called negative aspects of adjustment and well-being, such as anxiety, depression, poor mood, poor health, *etc.*, while others have focused on positive aspects such as optimism, satisfaction in life, better quality of living, positive mood, better physical health, *etc.* I want to discuss here which outcomes investigators have found to be related to the properties of the events we experience in our lives, again in light of the concept of personal control. These are major categories of event properties which we now know are related to positive and negative outcomes: (1) Event magnitude, (2) Event valence, (3) Event controllability, and (4) Event recurrence.

Event Magnitude

Major Life Events. By anybody's calculation, what happened to Jeff was major, life-changing, way beyond what one would ordinarily experience during the course of normal living. Its magnitude, its psychological impact, was far beyond a daily event such as getting a bill in your mail or you calling a friend. This distinction between these two general classes of events, small and routine or major and more rare, calls to our attention the large body of research on *event magnitude*. In addition to Jeff's event, other such large magnitude events would be getting married, getting divorced, buying a car, having a great overseas vacation, being placed in a nursing home, or losing a child. Note that such events are actually rare. Some major events are very undesirable, some are desirable, but in both cases they are unlikely to occur very often in your life. But when they do, they can cause significant disruption in our routine and our well-established habits which have helped us to get along in our accustomed style of living.

On the other hand, our lives are busy and filled with daily occurrences which are much smaller in magnitude than a major life event. Although these types of events are not as large in impact, there are many more of them and their cumulative effects may well add up to the same level of impact of major events. This is, of course, an empirical question, and later I will describe research which is focused on answering exactly that question.

I began this discussion of events by describing the story of Jeff Lewis and the major event that happened to him. Note, though, that in describing Jeff's experience, I used the phrase "happened to him." He was not in control of the behavior of the neighboring boy playing with the family gun and he had no way to prevent the accident from happening in the first place. So now I have made two major points about Jeff's experience: It was a major event as opposed to a small daily event, and it was uncontrollable, rather than controllable. But his experience calls up yet a third distinction that is important to our understanding of mental and physical health: The event's *valence*. It was obviously a very negative one; it was unpleasant, undesirable, and at least temporarily (in Jeff's case) it had a disruptive impact on what was otherwise a happy and productive life. Some events that are of large magnitude and out of our control are positive: Winning a lottery, for instance, or being given a large and unexpected raise at work are two positive experiences that are out of our control, they are large-impact, and they are desirable. (But look out for that lottery example; I will explain later why it is trickier than you might think.)

The story of how researchers and clinical practitioners came to look at the events of people's lives has an early beginning in the practice of psychiatry. Adolf Meyer, a Swiss-born psychiatrist moved to America and in the 1930s he became one of the leading psychiatrists of his day, including Presidency of the American Psychiatric Association. Although his approach to practice was basically medical, as is much of psychiatry, he proposed a fuller, more comprehensive approach to his practice. He engaged his "patients" more fully as people, not just a set of symptoms. He carefully interviewed them to get them to reveal as many aspects of their lives as he could, going beyond the medical/physiological aspects of their disorders. A key to this approach he discovered was to record the events of their lives in a "life chart" format which involved a detailed analysis of the number and types of events that they had experienced from childhood forward. Although this approach locates stress in the negative events that people experience, he also showed that even positive events can have stress-inducing effects.

The life chart model provided a key impetus for later investigators to refine and extend Meyer's basic methodology. This received its most sophisticated treatment in the landmark studies of Thomas Holmes and Richard Rahe.[1] To begin their investigation of events, they created a standardized list of 43 major, life-changing events, with "change" being the key concept. They defined an event as "a change from a previous state," and it is the change, *per se*, that is thought to be stressful; "readjustment required by the event" is another way of thinking about such events. Having created an initial large grouping of major events for their list, they then recruited a group of independent raters to score those events on the degree to which the event would require readjustment and also the length of time to accommodate to the event. Here are some examples selected from their final, now standardized list of 43 major life events, arranged in the degree of change required, from the highest (#1) down to a low degree of personal change required:

1. *Death of a spouse*
2. *Fired at work*
3. *Son or daughter leaving home*
4. *Trouble with boss*
5. *Vacation*
6. *Christmas*

Clearly Jeff Lewis experienced a "major life event" in this sense of the term.

Note that these are pretty infrequent events, but when they do happen to someone, they have a major impact on their well-being. Using this scale, researchers have been able to open up an entirely new kind of clinical science. The technique is to administer the Holmes and Rahe scale to a group of participants while also assessing their physical and mental well-being as correlated outcomes.

The results of a number of studies show that the more of these major events that one experiences in a given amount of time, the more likely that person will report greater levels of depression and anxiety.[2,3] Physical symptoms are also elevated when major events are experienced. Coronary heart attacks are significantly more likely to occur in patients who have been experiencing a significantly higher frequency of life stressors in the past 6 months.[4] Bereavement in terms of the loss of a significant other is related to reduced immune functioning, increasing one's risk of infection and illness.[5]

Other investigators saw the advantage of assessing specific types of major life events to determine their role in the well-being of various selected samples of participants. Among the somewhat more frequent major events in adults are retirement and relocation to another residence, often to a completely different city. For the former, Peter Peretti and Cedric Wilson[6] assessed the degree to which retirees felt high vs. low degrees of control over their retirement. Those who felt that they had little control over the retirement decision reported a lower quality of life than those who had felt more in control over the event. Along with retirement often comes relocation, a move to another home or another city. It is commonly thought that such an event is so disruptive that it would have negative consequences for adjustment. However, Richard Smith and Frederick Brand[7] found that such was not the case. Those people who rated that they had more voluntary choice in the move also reported better adjustment than those who reported that they had less freedom of choice in making the move. So the magnitude of the event, while still important to know, has to be seen in light of its controllability.

A common and certainly major life event is divorce. It is major, of course, because it puts a strain on our personal resources (financial, emotional, and social) while it requires a major shift and redirection in the life course of both partners. This disruption is stressful, not least because many of its aspects (financial, emotional, and social) but also because significant components of the overall experience are outside the controllability of the individual. Of particular significance in many cases is what happens after the divorce is finalized. Given that the legal side of the experience is completed, it is the post-divorce consequences that are important. Child visitation and upbringing arrangements have to be settled within the context of what the law requires, an external constraint on the freedom of the individual partners. These constraints apply to child visitation rights, child and spousal support laws, and these become key external causes of both partners' adjustment and well-being. These are often highly contentious and dissatisfaction with the arrangements can leads to serious noncompliance. However, Sanford Braver and his colleaues[8,9] have found that one key to satisfactory post-divorce arrangements is the degree to which the noncustodial parent feels some degree of personal control over the settlement. The more responsibility and personal control that the person feels in the settlement arrangements, the better the post-split involvement and continuing child support payments.

Remember back to the specific nature of the accident that happened to Jeff Lewis. His experience clearly is an example of a major life event, and it clearly undesirable, and it was a "change from a previous state." Note, though, that Jeff's outcome is clearly different from what much of the research data had been showing. That is why I am nesting this research into the broader context of personal mastery theory and research.

Mundane Daily Events. Major events have a big impact on us, and if and when they happen they are likely to make us undergo a life change. But they are infrequent; indeed, many people may experience only one or two of them throughout their entire adult life. We cannot get a very comprehensive picture of the adjustment and well-being of people if we have to rely on such infrequent occurrences. This issue of event magnitude animated some investigators to shift their focus from the rare events to the common events that are much more frequent in our lives. But since these events are very common and so typical of our daily living, at first glance one might not expect them to be of much significance in the overall scheme of understanding someone's mental health and well-being. But they can just as easily be thought of as "tipping points" in life where some people just suddenly snap after the occurrence of what would otherwise be thought of as a trivial event. Losing your car keys or having a shoelace break as you are rushing to an important appointment can be, in effect, devastating. It may well be that it is not the mere occurrence of some seemingly simple event but the cumulative effects of many such events over times and situations which gradually wear down our mental and physical resources.

Several research teams virtually simultaneously began this work soon after the initial burst of interest in the Holmes and Rahe approach. The two groups were at the University of California, Berkeley, where their initial report of results was published by Alan Kanner, James Coyne, Catherine Schaefer, and Richard Lazarus and the other team at Arizona State University involved myself and my colleagues Alex Zautra and Mary Davis. As you will see, a number of different techniques for assessing daily events have been developed, so in the discussion that follows I will present briefly the various techniques and findings in roughly the historical order in which they were published. I will make no attempt to cross-compare the various techniques; I present them as separate suggestions for you to think how the techniques, and their outcome results, might illuminate your own personal style of living.

The Kanner, *et al.* project[10] involved direct comparison of the effects of both major life events and small daily events on physical and mental well-being. Their project was pioneering in that it was the first major attempt to directly compare the outcomes of coping with both large-scale and smaller events. To do this, they had to think through what they meant by "small event," and this led them to develop the concept of "hassles" and "uplifts." They defined hassles as, *"irritants that can range from minor annoyances to fairly major pressures, problems, or difficulties."* They created a list of 117 of these. Here are some examples:

1. *Troublesome neighbors*
2. *Missing meals*
3. *Inconsiderate smokers*
4. *Someone owes you money*

They defined uplifts as: *"Uplifts are events that make you feel good. They can be sources of peace, satisfaction, or joy."* They generated a set of 135 of these. Here are some examples taken from their list:

1. *Practicing your hobby*
2. *Finding something presumed lost*
3. *Visiting, writing or phoning someone*
4. *Meeting your responsibilities*

Note that the experimenters did not formally assess the degree to which these events were controllable by the individual. I will return to this issue in a later part of this chapter. But they did test how these events' occurrences were related to measures of psychological well-being. They recruited a sample of 100 college students and adult community residents who answered their event questionnaires, indicating how often the event had occurred in the past month. These responses were correlated with the participants' responses to health and well-being questionnaires. Since each participant responded to both the major events of the Holmes and Rahe test and the hassles and uplifts scales, this allowed the experimenters to directly compare the effects of each on the outcome measures.

The results showed that the hassles' scores correlated with poorer health, but not with positive emotional feelings, whereas uplifts correlated with positive emotional feelings but not with poorer health and adjustment. The data allowed a statistical comparison of each set of events holding constant the other sets, allowing a test to see which was more significantly influential in the outcome measure. This type of analysis showed that the small events' measures had their effects *even when* statistically controlling for the occurrences of the major life events. Hassles were strongly correlated with the poorer health measure over and above the occurrence of the major life event. This is a particularly compelling result since major life event scores typically are considered to be causes of stress and negative outcomes. This is why a broken shoelace can cause such havoc. Since small events are so much more frequent in our daily living, this study confirms that they are a rich source of information about what kind of experiences are related to our physical and mental health, and they offer a better chance to help the person get more control over the patterns of their daily living.

Our research team at Arizona State University was independently developing our approach to event measurement with our "Index of Small Life Events" (ISLE).[11] Modeled closely on the methodology of the Holmes and Rahe technique, small daily items rated by independent judges as requiring less change in life were included in the list while making sure that events which were desirable and undesirable were specifically included in the listing. Some examples of these items are:

Observed a religious holiday
Went shopping for pleasure
Did poorly on an important test
Found a large unfavorable error in checkbook balance

We administered this scale and a number of mental health and well-being measures to samples of students and community-residing adults, correlating responses to the events' scale to the well-being scales. The results showed that people reporting higher amounts of undesirable events happening to them recently also reported feeling more demoralized, more distress, and negative emotions, and a poorer quality of life. Conversely, those who reported a greater number of positive small events reported higher feelings of well-being.

Again, in this study it was possible to compare the effects of small daily events to the effects of major life events. Theoretically, since daily events are so much more common than major events, one could argue that they would have their own set of effects independent of the effects of major events. The Kanner, *et al.* study's results supported that prediction. On the other hand, one could argue that since they are more common, we would have adapted to them and when stacked up against major events, they would not have any particularly important outcomes. In another study,[12] we administered the ISLE scale of small events, grouped together for their stressfulness, plus a separate measure of stressful major events to a large sample of 240 older adult community residents. They responded to our survey instruments once a month for 12 months, providing a dynamic, "moving picture" of their lives. Included in these monthly reports were questionnaires to measure mental health, particularly physical symptomatology and negative mood.

Statistical analyses examined for the relationships between both measures of events, daily and major, and measures of psychological distress.

The results showed that both classes of events, averaged over the monthly measures, were correlated with the poor adjustment measures. But these analyses allowed testing for each category of events controlling statistically for the frequency of occurrence of the other category. The results showed that even when removing the effects of the occurrence of major events, small daily events which were stressful were reliably related to the outcome measures of distress. Our data were in line with the Kanner, *et al.* results, so the effect is a robust one: Small daily events have a significant impact over time independently of major events we may have been experiencing.

Although I have been talking about major and small events as if they are separate entities, this is only for convenience of presentation. There is another important angle on this issue. Research by other investigators has shown that major events such as divorce or bereavement can lead to increases in smaller events that tend to follow up on such major disruptions. Divorce can lead to continuing conflicts with the spouse, and losing a spouse can lead to a greater burden of coping with the daily necessities of getting along.[13] You can get a cascading effect, making adjustment to smaller events more difficult to achieve. So these classes of events should not necessarily be thought of as disconnected or unrelated to each other. In your own life I am sure that you can easily come up with examples of a lot of nice things that followed up a major event such as getting a job or getting married, and a lot of undesirable things that followed getting a serious illness or being involved in a car wreck. We have to be aware of the interconnectedness of events.

Overall, then, the evidence from various studies suggests that the occurrence of small events plays a significant role in our well-being and that some of them may derive their influence by resulting from major stressors. Not all consequences need be thought of as negative, however, as Jeff Lewis's resilient response to his major life event shows so convincingly. He filled his life with resilient daily responses, controlling his daily events to enhance his resumption of the events he loved before his accident. In that sense, his golfing and public speaking are smaller events following after, and consequent upon, the one major event that shifted his entire life course.

Event Valence

Life is filled with desirable and undesirable events. Although they do vary in magnitude as we have just seen, it seems logical that their positive and negative properties might significantly weigh on how we judge the quality of our life, as well as on our mental and physical health. As basic, foundational information on the influence that events can have on us, Alex Zautra and I[14] reviewed the results of 17 separate studies in which the investigators examined the relationships between the frequency of experiencing positive and negative events and various measures of health and well-being. We found a high degree of consistency across the studies. Participants in those studies who reported experiencing relatively more desirable events in their lives also reported higher levels of psychological well-being, positive emotions, and life satisfaction. Completing the picture, those participants who reported experiencing more undesirable events also reported more psychological distress, more anxiety in their daily living, and higher levels of depression.

You might want to ask if there are any "cross-over" effects found in these studies. Is there a significant relationship between, say, desirable events and *negative* aspects of adjustment, and vice versa? Indeed, these studies did reveal that there is evidence for these more complex relationships. But it is particularly interesting that they are not precisely equal in direction of influence. For instance, the frequency of occurrence of desirable events was not related to negative aspects of adjustment. But in fact experiencing greater amounts of undesirable events not only correlated with the negative aspects of adjustment but also tended to suppress the more positive aspects of well-being. This asymmetry in the effects of events is a major consideration in many areas of psychological research and clinical practice, but to cover that issue extensively would take us astray from the main points I want to make here. Interested readers may wish to pursue this issue by reading research articles by our team of researchers[15,16,17] and other investigators.[18]

Finally, there is logically another aspect of small events that deserves deeper consideration. In spite of all of the attention given to desirable and undesirable events, some possibly significant amounts of our daily living are connected with very mundane events which are *neutral* in tone and tend not to engage our positive or negative motivations. Our attention is usually focused on the more emotionally positive and negative aspects of our daily living. But if we do actually cause these neutral events to occur (tying your shoelace, choosing a red dress to wear) or if they arise outside of our control (a green light changes to red, your mail is delivered), your response to them automatically reflects your ability to manage your life. Lacking success in managing the small things in life can be quite devastating. They may be neutral in tone, but your actions or reactions to them can have positive benefits for you because they present an occasion for you to exercise your personal mastery in handling them. There is a hidden personal causation property to these otherwise apparently uninteresting events; they set the stage and provide opportunities for exercising your personal mastery. I want to elaborate on this point in the following section.

Event Controllability

An astute reader will by now have noticed something going on that researchers had not yet explicitly noted. If you look at the examples of events I listed, there seems to be a natural tendency for "hassles" to be more negative in their emotional tone, while "uplifts" and "desires" tend to be positive in their emotional tone. But something else appears to be operating in those lists. Hassles appear to be those events which "happen" to us, arising from outside of us, while uplifts appear to be more often caused by the person's own desires, initiatives, and activities.

If these suspicions are accurate, that implies that there is something inherently positive about being in control over the events of your life and there is something inherently stressful and negative about experiencing events over which you have no control. So if you will take a personal mastery approach you can see that event valence really cannot be understood very well without considering the cause of the event; controllability is the key to event impact, either for major events or small daily events. If you will recall those lists of events that I presented in the Introduction, you can now see that this issue was the underpinning of the way I constructed those lists...

Our ASU research team raised that issue in the research project I described above.[11] In addition to having our independent group of judges score the small events on their desirability/undesirability, we also had them rate the items on the basis of how *controllable* by the individual they were. The instructions to our judges indicated to them that they were to rate each event on a 5-point scale of the extent to which a person could, if they wished, prevent the event from happening (1) on up to rate how much a person could make an event such as this one happen (5).

Our assumptions were confirmed. When we analyzed the responses of our judges, we found that desirable events were much more likely to be rated as controllable; 70% of the time they were rated as controllable while they were rated as uncontrollable only 9% of the time. Undesirable events were more mixed in their ratings, but more than half again as many were rated as uncontrollable as were rated controllable. This connection makes entirely good sense; we tend to pursue and "make it happen" desirable events; undesirable events are much murkier in terms of their causation.

We then administered these items to a sample of 113 college students along with measures of their quality of life and several aspects of their mental health. The results showed what we predicted: Participants reporting having a greater amount of controllable positive events also reported higher levels of their quality of life and better mental health than those who reported fewer such experiences. Those who had experienced greater numbers of uncontrollable negative events reported poorer quality of life and poorer mental health.

So in a linked series of studies our team systematically began a series of studies investigating the effects of the occurrence of small daily events from the perspective of their controllability. As I shall show later in this section, there is a hidden "reverse factor" operating here: All other things held constant, things we personally cause tend to make us feel good, and things that "happen to us," events we do not ourselves cause, tend to be negative in their impact. This is a more complicated picture, involving both positive and negative event properties as discovered by Kanner, *et al.*, and personal mastery factors as we showed. We wanted to pursue this issue and we systematically went one more step to get an answer to it.

Our investigation of this issue followed standard event-checking methodology, but we carefully pre-tested the events to be included in our list for their degree of how much the person could cause them to occur. We had two ideas already published in organizational and psychological research which we found to be highly useful in thinking about this issue. First was the pioneering work of Fredrick Herzberg. Some of his pathbreaking works were already well known, with *Work and the Nature of Man* having a major impact in the intersection between worker psychology and motivation research.[19] American business had become greatly concerned with worker productivity, and Herzberg was widely sought out for his consultation on issues of worker motivation.

In his "motivation-hygiene theory," Herzberg distinguished between two very different mechanisms which relate to productivity. What he called "hygiene factors" are external, physical and environmental factors set up by management to increase worker efficiency and productivity. They arrange workplace conditions such as more work space, cleanliness, better lighting, they can monitor the adequacy of workplace technical arrangements, pay, benefits, *etc*. These are obvious things that management can do, and they do them for the purpose for influencing workers' activities.

Working with hygiene factors seems a quite obvious mechanism to change worker productivity, but Herzberg had a much more sophisticated and realistic model of human behavior. His argument was that workers have basic workplace needs which can be met by adequate work-environment arrangements, but as human beings they have psychological needs as well. This is an entirely different approach, and these psychological needs operate in a completely different manner. He recognized that we all have basic needs to be valued, to have a sense of achievement, to feel competent and responsible, and to advance and grow. He calls these "motivator factors" as opposed to his hygiene factors. His model requires enriching the work experience by opening up more avenues for personal achievement, supporting a sense of being valued, and encouraging individual creativity. Changing hygiene factors misses this critical distinction. In fact, his many studies on organizations showed that the two sets of factors are independent of each other. Improving hygiene factors can reduce dissatisfaction but will not increase satisfaction; these are different domains of motivation. Herzberg created the concept of KITA ("Kick in the a...") as a prime example of how employers can get compliant workers by threats and other forms of hygiene factors which may increase productivity but come at the cost of high levels of dissatisfaction on the motivator side of the equation.

The key distinction for us in the Herzberg two-factor approach was the great emphasis he placed on workers' sense of achievement, responsibility, and personal growth. These are natural consequences of being able to control your own environment. Our personal mastery approach slightly reinterprets Herzberg's model: While any job has its necessary requirements, giving workers freedom to exercise their own initiative and enhancing the sense that what they do on the job actually reflects their personal control, we would expect that it would improve their satisfaction and productivity.

We had a second line of research available to us as we began our studies. In the realm of studies on human motivation, Richard DeCharms[20] had coined the concepts of "origin" and "pawn." Although DeCharms's original ideas were developed to apply as personality or trait descriptions of people, his ideas about being an active agent in one's life, an "origin" or a passive recipient of experiences, a "pawn," beautifully described what we were wanting to study in finding out how people's well-being is related to their daily experiences. We took his ideas of originness and pawnness and used them to characterize daily events taken from standard event-listing methodology. To do this, we again had an independent group of raters check the extent to which items we selected from various lists involved some action by the person's own skills and efforts and other items having just the opposite properties. Also, of course, we had the event items rated for their valence, their positivity or their negativity.

This category system then led us to create a 40-item event checklist.[21] Positive events are easily thought of as being either something that we choose to do (Origin events) or good things that happen to us (Pawn events). Since most people most of the time do not deliberately inflict negative things on themselves, the nature of causation for them would be more ambiguous, so the "origin" part of negative events is hard to imagine. So for the sake of simplicity and clarity, we combined all negative events into one category, and considered them as providing useful comparison information for our results on the Origin-Pawn distinction we could more easily make for positive events. Here are some examples of the 3 categories of items and examples that we used in our study of well-being:

10 Positive Origin (PO) events:
An outstanding personal achievement
Beginning to date
Increase in number of friendships

10 Positive Pawn (PP) events:
Reduction in course requirements
Increase in the number of compliments received from others
Given increased freedom from restrictions

20 Negative Events (NO + NP) events:
Personal rejection by a close friend
Loss of a close friend
Decrease in ability to get along with others

In our research project we presented these events (without, of course, revealing their valence or cause designation) to a sample of 148 college students, along with a battery of standard measures of quality of life and mental health measures. The results again fit the pattern I have described in other studies using these methods, but we also found some intriguing results. As you might expect, Positive Origin events correlated well with high quality of life while both classes of negative events were related to poorer mental health and a lower quality of life. Again, and as you might expect, experiencing both Origin and Pawn events which were negative led to poorer quality of life and poorer mental health. In this case, negativity effects swamped out personal causation feelings.

But now for a more intriguing finding. Positive *pawn* events also related to poorer mental health! To experience positive events, but ones over which you had no personal control, was shown to be related to poorer adjustment. This was true also of negative pawn events, so it is "pawnness" per se and not the positive or negative valence of our daily events that leads us to have poorer feelings overall.

We confirmed this finding in a later study[22] in which we found, in a sample of rheumatoid arthritis patients, that while positive controllable events were related to greater positive feelings and reduced negative feelings, positive pawn events also tended to be related to increased *negative* feelings. Apparently the fact that you have experienced a positive event, although it may be related to positive feelings, also is related to more negative feelings; the fact that the events were out of the person's personal control tended to generate mixed feelings, in terms of increasing both positive and negative feelings. Zautra and I coined the phrase, "stressful highs" to account for the fact that the events can be positive in valence but stressful because they arise from outside of our personal control.

The drive to be in control of the daily events of one's life is indeed a major motivation in life, and being in a context where events are outside of your control, even positive ones, suggests the unfortunate effects of loss of control. Although at first it may seem unlikely to you, there are studies on lottery winners which confirm this finding. You might at first glance assume that winning a lottery would be a wonderful experience, but many studies suggest otherwise. I will discuss those studies in Chapter 5.

In another project exploring the connection between controllability and event valence,[23] we developed another formulation of what is involved when an event is thought of as arising from the personal control motivations of the person *vs.* events which arise from outside of the person's personal causation. We gave these classes of events handy names: We called the list of events under one's personal control "desires," and the events which arise outside of our control and which put pressure on us to be resolved "demands." We developed a set of 100 of these demand and desire events (50 of each) based on their desirability and controllability. We found a great deal of agreement among our judges, over 80%, giving us confidence in our original thinking about these event properties. Here are some examples of Demand and Desire events:

Demand Events	Desire Events
Refrigerator needed cleaning	*Swimming*
Needed to find a babysitter	*Going to church*
Car needed gas/oil	*Dating*
Had to prepare meals	*Eating a favorite food*

We administered these lists to college students in one sampling and community-residing adults in another sampling. We developed separate tests of events for each group in order to assess more carefully the "event ecologies" of their daily living. We then recruited samples of adults and college student volunteers to help us test the relationships between event occurrences and outcome measures of well-being. In addition to reporting on how many demand and desire events they had been experiencing in the past two weeks, both samples also responded to standard measures of quality of life and positive and negative mood scales to assess their feelings over the same past two-week period. Since we have shown that positive and negative aspects of moods, emotions, and well-being are generally independent of each other, we treated the scores of each type of adjustment separately to correlate them with how many demands and desires they had been experiencing.

As we expected, and for both samples of participants, the greater the number of demand events the participants had been experiencing was related to more negative mood and a general lower quality of life. Conversely, having more desire events was correlated with higher positive mood and higher quality of life. Our data revealed that not only is event magnitude important to our well-being, in this case small daily events, the data also show, equally importantly, that the causal properties of events give them their importance for our well-being.

Responding to Our Events

Of course we run our lives with more action than just having an event occur to us, or causing one. We also respond to them, and our responses have consequences. My colleagues Michael McCall, Robert Grossman, Alex Zautra, and Charles Guarnaccia[24] recognized this possibility by making our measurement technique more sensitive and comprehensive by assessing all three components of an event experience. In another sample of participants, in this case a large sample of 101 college students, we asked them to report at the end of the day for 4 successive days: (1) if an event (demand or desire) had arisen during the day, (2) if it had, did they actually respond to it and, if they did, (3) how satisfied were they with the outcome of the sequence. Again, we assessed their feelings of positive and negative mood, their perceived quality of life, and other measures of well-being.

The results of this more comprehensive assessment of the effects of daily events agreed with the results of our previous studies, but with additional insights. The number of demands that people experienced was related to poorer health reports and lower quality of life, as you might expect. But when the participants reported greater activity at actually *dealing* with those demands, they then reported better health and better quality of life. Even more interesting, the more satisfied people were with their coping with those demands, the "outcome satisfaction" measure, we saw improved reports of health and quality of life.

So while the number of demands pressuring us results in more negative consequences, actually becoming active and doing something about them and being satisfied with the outcome of those coping efforts was shown to reduce the negative effects we might otherwise find. For this particular sample of college students, the number of desire events was relatively small, less than the number of demand events. Not surprisingly, the amount of desire event activity and satisfaction with the outcome of that activity related to positive mood. Overall, it appears that this particular sample of college students was busily engaged in coping with their school activities which acted as demand events, and they had little time to put aside to experience desirable activities.

Bringing in this additional aspect of event control, measuring how much effort and actions we actually expend on demands and desires gives us a much more complete picture of the how events fit in with our daily activities. From what I have said so far, it is obvious that we need to consider not only event magnitude and event valence, but the apparently tight connection between event desirability/undesirability and controllability. That requires a more complex type of study, but the connection appears to be a tight one. We infused this type of thinking in our experimental personal mastery intervention project which I will discuss in Chapter 9.

Our study's focus on daily event controllability has a therapeutic implication. Dealing with events once they have arisen may seem truly like a hassle as Kanner, *et al.* studied, but from a personal mastery perspective they are a golden opportunity to expand our capacities and outlook on life.

They are small in magnitude and they can be handled if we are motivated to take them on and deal with them, rather than letting them hang in our lives, putting pressure on us to get resolved. The American philosopher/psychologist William James has stated it beautifully:

> *Keep the faculty of effort alive in you by a little gratuitous exercise every day. That is, be systematically heroic in little unnecessary points, do every day or two something for no other reason than its difficulty, so that, when the hour of dire need draws nigh, it may find you not unnerved or untrained to stand the test. Asceticism of this sort is like the insurance which a man pays on his house and goods. The text does him no good at the time, and possibly may never bring him a return. But if the fire does come, his having paid it will be his salvation from ruin. So with the man who had daily inured himself to habits of concentrated attention, energetic volition, and self-denial in unnecessary things. He will stand like a tower when everything rocks around him, and his softer fellowmortals are winnowed like chaff in the blast.*[25]

Event Recurrence

Continuing with our review of event properties, there is one more property of events that requires special discussion: Their *recurrence,* their chronicity or repetitive frequency of occurrence. Some events are one-time occurrences, such as the wounding of Jeff Lewis, whereas other events are highly frequent and even regularly recurrent, such as going to work every day. While investigators typically estimate event frequency by counting up how many events from a given list a participant reports experiencing, this dimension of recurrence is specific to each event; how many times does a particular event occur in a person's life in a given time period? For instance, "getting a flat tire" is usually non-recurrent although it may have negative consequences for our well-being. But "having an upset stomach" time and time again is a very different matter. "Play cards with friends every Saturday night" is a recurrent positive event, and the question is, does it have a more beneficial effect than "had an unexpected birthday party," which is basically non-recurrent within at least a year's time frame? Experiencing a divorce can have unrelenting, chronic consequences long after the separation... or of course it could have recurring positive outcomes as well.

This distinction between recurrent and non-recurrent events clearly raises important considerations from a control perspective. If an event is recurrent, then we can predict it or anticipate it. Suzanne Thompson[26] reviewed a number of studies on how we react to aversive events such as misfortunes and injuries such as those that cause us pain and stress. She finds that one of the key dimensions in our ability to withstand such events is their predictability and our own personal estimates of our ability to endure them. If they are planned and if we believe that we can control them effectively, then we will have less anxiety and more ability to deal with them. I think that the title of her article captures very well the essence of her findings: "Will It Hurt Less If I Can Control It? A Complex Answer To A Simple Question."

The issue of predictability is part of event recurrence or chronicity. In a study of of 246 community-residing adults, Alex Zautra, Charles Guarnaccia and I[27] categorized their event reports into, among other categories, recurrent and non-recurrent small daily events (again using the ISLE reporting instrument). The results showed that recurring health events were significantly correlated with higher anxiety and depression scores, presumably because they were not controllable events and were going to keep on recurring. The results of a study of families under stress such as recent bereavement, child illness, and divorce, reported many more recurrent stressors than comparable control families without such stressors.[13] These families reported an average of 10 recurrent stressors in the past month. They also reported significantly higher levels of anxiety and sadness compared to controls who did not report such high levels of recurrent stressors in their lives. Those major events of bereavement, and childhood illness, and divorce have disrupted the lives of those parents, rendering them susceptible to the occurrence of more small but stressful daily events which, in turn, become recurring stresses in their lives. This shows again that, in our environment of events, such occurrences are often intertwined sometimes leading to a cascade of events which spin off of one event, particularly a recurring one.

One way that investigators study the recurrence property of life events is to review the findings from national quality of life surveys, where events are now commonly assessed. Such surveys are becoming more common and we are getting valuable insights into the lifestyles of residents who were selected for being interviewed, usually on a random sampling basis. One particularly valuable feature of these surveys is that they often involve repeated surveying, assessing the participants' responses several times over a significant span of time, often covering a span of years.

One such analysis of a survey in Germany by Maike Luhmann and Michael Eid[28] studied the effects of three kinds of multiple occurrence events: Becoming unemployed more than once, getting divorced more than once, and getting married more than once. The results showed that life satisfaction decreases after a second bout of becoming unemployed, whereas life satisfaction increases after a second divorce. Remarriage tends to have no particularly prominent effects on life satisfaction. Interestingly, repeated recurrences of all types of events were related to decreases in life satisfaction compared to single occurrences of the other types of events. Clearly, then, if we want to have a more complete picture of life satisfaction, we have to make an attempt to get repeated judgments from the person over time to look for the effects of chronic occurrences. With repetition, we have a better chance to detect personal control capabilities or situations in which we suffer the consequences of experiencing events over which we have no control, such as unemployment.

In a study of undergraduates, Mark Wright, Alex Zautra, and Sanford Braver[29] showed that the outcomes of recurrent events are rated by the participants as being more personally controllable than nonrecurring events. This may be one reason why chronic health conditions such as arthritis, cancer, and heart problems (major events) and smaller daily events such as a stomach ache or recurrent headaches have such damaging effects on our well-being; it depends on their controllability. While their magnitude is an important consideration, and while their valence (undesirable in this case) is also important, the fact that the event is going to occur over and over when you cannot control it is a key to their harmful consequences. On the other hand, knowing that the event is going to occur allows you to be able to anticipate the occurrence and prepare your reactions to it. The Wright, Zautra, and Braver data in fact show that recurrent events are rated as more under a person's control than nonrecurrent events. In the language of Fred Rothbaum, John Weisz, and Samuel Snyder[30] *predictability* is its own form of control, and research evidence they cite supports a model where this form of control is related to improved adjustment and well-being.

In understanding our world well enough to be able to predict event occurrences in our daily life, we are well on our way to being able to adjust to that world even when the events it brings us may be undesirable ones. With his new prosthetic devices, Jeff Lewis was again able to predict and therefore bring the events of his life under his own personal control, an exercise of his personal mastery of his life, with obviously positive benefits.

A Surprising Conclusion

In this chapter I have reviewed a broad range of events that we experience in life, exploring their properties that are important from a personal control perspective: Their magnitude, their valence, their controllability, and their chronicity. I particularly noted that, independent of event magnitude, there is a strong connection between event valence and controllability: Most of our self-caused events tend to be positive or desirable, while events arising from forces outside of us are more commonly undesirable, although of course there are many exceptions to both "rules." What I particularly wanted to point out is the third category which does not receive much attention: Small, daily events that are not necessarily either desirable or undesirable. So much of our life is filled with these routine experiences, but from a personal mastery perspective, they can be a goldmine of strength for our mental health: They provide for us a myriad of ways to assert our mastery when we make them occur, and we can avoid hassles and problems in our lives handling them when they arise from outside forces. In many ways, it is the "undone task" that is the constant bane of our busy modern lives. As "Shorty," one of my dairy plant co-workers told me many years ago, "If you can't do what you want to do, then you gotta do what you have to do." Asserting our mastery of more neutral, routine experiences nevertheless give us boundless opportunities for asserting our mastery if we can see them as opportunities rather than burdens.

Upcoming Topics

I am devoting the next two chapters to a review of the evidence on the properties of events and their consequences for our well-being. In the next chapter, 4, I will review the properties of undesirable events and what studies show about their outcomes for us. In the chapter following that, 5, I will discuss the properties of desirable events and their consequences for us. You may find yourself surprised about some of these results (for instance, you may experience less desire to enter lotteries!).

Of course, this particular science of your personal mastery beliefs and their consequences has to be made specific to you, the individual reader. So, again as I said in my Preface, I encourage you to apply "interactive reading" as you see and interpret the results of the studies I am presenting. While the specific examples of events may apply only some of the time in your daily living, the underlying principles are applicable to all of our lives.

Chapter 4

Undesirable Events Can Threaten Mastery

In the grand scheme of life, people seek a good life with as many desirable events and as few undesirable events as possible. Regardless of the wisdom of that life choice, the personal mastery perspective suggests that there is one key consideration in how this lifestyle condition is to come about; knowing the difference between events that we personally cause to occur, and those that arise outside of our own personal control. This is a more refined template for our lives as stated in the Serenity Prayer I presented in the Preface.

This event-based approach to "things" is different from other approaches to people's lives, such as an economic one that investigates their wealth or poverty, or such as a religious one, that investigates their belief or disbelief in a higher power, or from a political one that reveals their preference for a particular political party, *etc.* There are many ways to categorize and study people, but by focusing on events the personal mastery approach is particularly productive because it cuts across all of those aspects of a person's life; it provides a comprehensive approach to the psychological dynamics underlying the way we match our inner recourses and motivations with the world of events in which we live.

My discussion of the properties of events in Chapter 3 gave us a good start on understanding how you can experience more satisfaction with events as they occur in your life, both self-caused and externally caused. But there is much more to say about what researchers have discovered. In the next two chapters I will intensify my review by focusing on the two key ways in which undesirable and desirable events occur. We now know that "occurrence" can either be by accident, an external cause such as that experienced by Jeff Lewis, or it can be an event that arises from deliberate, intentional causation by some person.

In this chapter, I want to use our personal mastery approach to show the effects of undesirable experiences, when things go badly and the person has their sense of control threatened. It can be a devastating experience. In the chapter following this one, devoted to desirable events, we will see how this can have beneficial effects for us. But, again, we can have such events arising "accidentally" and those caused either by the person or by someone else. In this perhaps unusual perspective, even seemingly desirable events can have undesirable consequences.

Our Perceived Responsibility for Undesirable Events

Note that I have not yet discussed one particular category of events: Negative, undesirable events that we personally cause to occur. Since usually people are not motivated to make themselves unhappy by deliberately causing themselves to experience undesirable events, this category of possible occurrences is not an extensively-investigated issue. These are commonly and nonscientifically called "mistakes" or "errors." Naturally we generally do not think of this type of negative event as caused by our intention or deliberate causation. But these things happen, and it is instructive for our understanding of personal control in all of its facets. A very careful and detailed study of these events was reported by John Mirowsky and Catherine Ross.[1] They conducted a telephone interview of 809 Chicago residents, asking a set of questions assessing the extent to which they accepted personal responsibility for desirable and undesirable events or denied responsibility, blaming bad luck or external forces for undesirable events. The results of the residents' causal explanations were then correlated with a standard measure of feelings of depression.

Several findings are of interest here. First, most people said that they were the cause of *both* desirable and undesirable events: Blaming external causes was much less frequent. And that same pattern of explanations was related to lower depressive feelings. So accepting responsibility as reflected in questions like these, "My misfortunes are the result of mistakes I have made" and "I am responsible for my failures" are in fact correlated with less depressive feelings. Ask you might expect, the desirable event items such as "I am responsible for my own successes" and "I can do just about anything I really set my mind to" are also related to less depressive thinking. Beliefs in one's control trumps event negativity. So, considered from both angles of desirable and undesirable event causation, personal control beliefs are the key to better mental health. I will return to this same effect later in the chapter in describing research on unquestionably externally caused events such as rape.

On the other hand, of course we are distinctly motivated to cause our own desirable events and to avoid undesirable ones. In this chapter I want to focus on conditions in which our sense of personal master is threatened by negative events. In the next chapter I will turn our attention to positive events.

When Our Sense of Control is Threatened by the Environment

There are occasions and situations in life in which our freedom to exercise our personal choice is threatened or even eliminated. Sometimes this happens as the result of an accident, such as happened to Jeff Lewis. In fact, a definition of the term "accident" makes some useful distinctions. I found the following definition at: http://www.thefreedictionary.com

Accident: An unexpected and undesirable event, especially one resulting in damage or harm

This definition certainly characterizes Jeff's story. Since we are dealing with "unexpected" causes, then one's personal control beliefs are undermined by the lack of foresight and planning which usually characterize our life. The boy who shot Jeff surely did not have intentions to harm in mind when he started playing with the gun. But there are also negative events which "happen" which do not arise by chance but by *deliberate* intention of some else. Rape is a terrible example of this type of occurrence. It is a negative event but it is not accidental; it was planned by someone who had harmful intentions. Psychologists have studied responses to various types of accidents and to accidental or deliberate harm. I will discuss examples of each of these in turn.

Accidents as Externally-Caused Undesirable Events

There is virtually no way for Jeff or anyone else to think that he was an active cause of his accident. But in other cases causality may not be so clear-cut. It is important that people maintain their sense of mastery when it is threatened, but their perceptions of the circumstances of the occurrence of undesirable events have some surprising subtleties. There are a number of angles on how this occurs.

In one of the original studies of this kind of experience, the focus was on accidents resulting in paraplegia and quadriplegia. These accidents mirror closely what happened to Jeff Lewis, so they can provide information for us to better understand Jeff's incident. Drs. Ronnie Janoff-Bulman and Camille Wortman[2] interviewed a group of 29 spinal cord injury patents at the Rehabilitation Institute of Chicago, Illinois. These patients were mostly young males in their 20s and 30s, all of whom had been rendered paraplegic or quadriplegic by an injury in the past year. They had experienced such major negative life events as an automobile accident, a private plane or motorcycle crash, a barn or building construction accident, and a high school football accident. These active, healthy young men, busily going about the tasks and pleasures of life (demands and desires, in our languages) experienced a serious accident and were suddenly paralyzed, in all likelihood for the rest of their lives. How does the human mind handle this type of catastrophe?

I am interested in the control-related consequences of this type of experience for what we can learn about threats to our sense of well-being. The investigators conducted in-depth interviews with the patients, asking a number of probing question about what they, the patients, thought was the cause of their accident. The investigators also asked broader questions about the patients' adjustment, their well-being, their sense of optimism and their general outlook on the future. In addition, Janoff-Bulman and Wortman interviewed the nurses and social workers who were dealing with the patients on a daily basis. With all of these measures, they had good grounds for judging how well the patients were adjusting to their condition.

The "cause" questions that they asked the patients concerned such aspects as how much self-blame they felt, how avoidable they thought that the accident was, how much other people or the environment caused the accident, and how much luck or just sheer chance caused it ("bad luck"). These questions were intended to assess the patients' perceptions of the internal or external cause of their experience. Then the investigators could relate that cause information to the information on the patients' adjustment provided by the staff. The results indicated that there were in fact two types of patients' explanations resulting in two distinct categories of adjustment to the accident: "Good copers" and "poor copers." Good copers were those patients who were more resilient in that they had a positive attitude toward their physical therapy, they were working hard toward improving their physical abilities, and they wanted to be independent. Poor copers were those patients who were denying the degree of their disability, they expected to get better without any great effort on their part, and they showed no particular interest in working on their rehabilitation exercises.

On the basis of what you now know of personal mastery and control motivation, what would you think the connection with personal control beliefs would be between these two sets of measures on these patients? Those patients who were categorized as good copers were those who *blamed themselves* for their accident! The good copers where those who saw the causation of their accident as due to their own behavior or to their lack of foresight and not paying enough attention to the dangers that their activities had created. Those patients who were categorized as poor copers blamed other people or back luck for their accidents; they were focused on the lack of justice in their world or they were angry at other people for having caused their misfortune.

These results may at first be surprising: Why would blaming oneself for a bad outcome be a positive, healthy way to think about this experience? Is not the mind supposed to assert control over good outcomes and deny responsibility for bad outcomes? The key to this apparent dilemma is contained in one additional question that the investigators asked: They asked the patients how much they felt that they could have *avoided* the accident. The results showed that those patients who were better copers felt that they could not have avoided the accident. The poor copers felt that that they could have avoided the accident.

So here we have been given a good insight into the power of beliefs in personal control, and the results were exactly in line with what we would expect from the study by Mirowsky and Ross that I discussed earlier in this chapter. The good copers accepted *responsibility* for their accident; they saw it as a consequence of their own freely chosen behavior. That *free choice* was the key to their better well-being. Just feeling that they were in control of what happened to them, even though it was very negative, enabled them to develop better adjustment to their situation. It may be easier to grasp the personal control principles operating in this situation if you think about the mental processes of the poor copers. Here is someone whose formerly active lifestyle essentially has been destroyed because, in their mind, of the actions of some other person, someone outside of their own personal control or, perhaps worse, of this mysterious, uncontrollable external cause called "bad luck." Life got "out of control" and they were the passive, helpless victim of it. Thinking that the accident could have been avoided leaves them with the counterfactual "if only…" regretful way of thinking.

Resigning yourself to a fate such as this is, in its own way, a form of believing in your own personal control. Here is a quote from one of the good copers:

…we were engaged in a contact sport. We both were doing something that we wanted to do. Really, I don't think I could have avoided it.

Resigning yourself to an unavoidable experience is a way of asserting your own control over your feelings and your responses. To pass causation over to external forces is to acknowledge your uncontrollability and a lack of mastery over your experiences.

Of course, these results are in no way a recommendation that one should invariably take responsibility for bad outcomes. But you will recall Jeff Lewis's personal motto that "don't let things you can't do stop you from doing the things you can do." That is basically a statement of mental optimism and resilience in the face of negative experiences, but the focus is also on taking control of your life even with serious restrictions. That is a very different picture from the image we have of the poor copers, blaming others and finding no helpful way out of the thought that one had no control over one's own fate, and "nothing can be done about it."

Chronic Physical Pain as an Externally-Caused Undesirable Event

There is another category of bad things that "happen" but do not have any clear connection to either something that the person does or to something that someone else does. This is the category of event experiences involving disease, illness, and sickness. Unless someone with an illness has particularly bad habits, they would not be considered as having "caused" their illness. Psychologists and medical researchers have developed an entire field of research and practice surrounding poor health and what physicians and the individual can do about it. This discipline is called *health psychology*. A significant body of investigation in this tradition has dealt with personal control issues and their role in sickness and health. I want to discuss how control issues play an important role in how we experience negative health events and how thinking in control terms can help us to understand more effective ways for recovery.

Glenn Affleck, Howard Tennen, Carol Pfeiffer, and Judith Fifield[3] at the University of Connecticut School of Medicine enlisted a sample of 92 rheumatoid arthritis patients to respond to questionnaires about their illness. That choice of this particular illness was quite deliberate. Rheumatoid arthritis is a chronic autoimmune disease causing inflammation and pain in the joints and musculature. It is painful, progressive, incurable, it is not personally controllable by the patient, and medicines are often only partially effective in easing patients' pain. One particularly negative aspect of it is the sudden flare-ups of inflammation which are unpredictable. From our control perspective, the recurrence, unexpectedness and uncontrollability make it a particularly destructive disorder because the person did not deliberately cause it, and they cannot even predict when their pain will flare-up. But the fact that it is basically incurable means that personal mastery motivations really cannot be effective in eliminating the disease.

The investigators asked their patients an extensive set of questions about their illness, and combined their responses to those questions with medical data from the physician and nurse practitioners to gauge illness severity and the patients' adjustment to their illness. To analyze patients' own personal understanding of and reactions to their disease, the investigators' questions probed control issues: How much control the patient felt over their day-to-day symptoms, over the future course of their disease, and over the medical care and treatment of their illness.

The results showed that the patients were well able to distinguish the various forms of control. They felt that they had more control over their *symptoms* than they did over the course of the actual disease itself. That made a difference in their adjustment; their feelings of having some personal control over their symptoms were related to better adjustment. Since in fact we do have at least some ability to deal with and even partially control our reactions to our symptoms, then this result is in line with what we would expect from applying a personal mastery perspective to this debilitating disease. However, and equally important, if the patients felt that they could actually control the *course* of the disease itself, then that was related to poorer adjustment. In any real sense, a patient cannot control the way rheumatoid arthritis develops, but the more that patients rated that they believed that they could control it, the worse their adjustment. A similar positive effect was found for their ratings of their control over the medical care and treatment; those who reported that they had more control over these aspects of their illness also reported more positive forms of adjustment. This distinction between the unchangeable nature of the disease itself and the changeable nature of how we deal with our symptoms provides a key insight into how we can infuse personal control thinking in medical settings.

Perry Nicassio, a leading researcher of arthritis and his colleagues Kenneth Wallston, Leigh Callahan, Marianne Herbert, and Theodore Pincus saw the value of that model for studying the psychological consequences of arthritis.[4] They developed a psychometric instrument for studying the mental health and functional health of rheumatoid arthritis patients. They called it "The Arthritis Helplessness Index" (AHI), a 15-item scale to which arthritis patients were to respond with 4-choice answers from "Strongly Agree" to "Strongly Disagree." Here is a sample of some of the items:

> *Arthritis is controlling my life.*
> *Managing my arthritis is largely my own responsibility.*
> *No matter what I do, or how hard I try, I just can't seem to get relief from my arthritis.*
> *I am coping effectively with my arthritis.*
> *It seems as though fate and other factors beyond my control affect my arthritis.*

Studying a sample of 219 RA patients, they found that participants reporting greater helplessness reported feeling lower self-esteem, greater depression and anxiety, and poorer ability to handle their daily activities. But a higher belief in being able to control their arthritis symptoms was an effective correlate of better adjustment to their illness. This study set off a round of additional studies extending the use of the AHI to other outcome measures, but the core finding remained: One can get better adaptation to this destructive disease by developing a better sense of one's ability to control your reactions to it.

Cancer

Cancer is an unfortunately widespread and certainly a personally uncontrollable disease. One of the most debilitating of all chronic diseases, cancer is the observable result of a multifaceted set of cellular abnormalities. It is now the dominant concern in medical research and public policy because of its still-mysterious causes and uncertain course of treatment success. Not only is the disease itself a threat to one's sense of being in control of the events in one's life, but treatment regimens also require the patient to give over control to highly-trained specialists who in turn require a high degree of compliance from the patient during the sometimes quite extended and exhausting treatment phase. Although great progress is being made almost daily in diagnosis and treatment of this illness in its many forms, from our perspective, it represents a serious threat to a person's sense of personal mastery and control. Treatment requires the person to rely on others, the treatment team. Again, we have here an example of "vicarious control" as we saw in the work of Affleck, *et al.* and rheumatoid arthritis patients.

In a study of 55 cancer patients, Shelly Taylor, Vicki Helgeson, Geoffrey Reed, and Laurie Skokan[5] asked patients about their perceptions of control over the cancer being asserted by their physicians. The results showed that the patients' own physical condition was an important modifier of how they reacted to being "controlled" in the sense we use it here: Control of the cancer treatment is taken on by the physician, not the patient. The investigators' results showed that when the patient had a good prognosis and treatment was going well, then believing that others (physicians) had control over the disease was related to better psychological adjustment. That is, patients were much better off when they felt that doctors and nurses were going to have control over curing their disease when the illness was in fact improving. However, when the prognosis was poor and it looked like things were going to get worse, believing in vicarious control was related to *poorer* adjustment. Control by external forces such as physicians is a positive force for good when there is a good chance that their efforts will pay off in better health for you; it means relying on other people whom you can trust, so dependency on other people is not necessarily a bad condition. But when things are not going to go well and the efforts of others look like they will not be successful, then being forced medically to have to depend on them means a loss of control and consequently poor mental health outcomes.

These results neatly confirm what has been found for control processes in arthritis patients. Coping and adjustment are enhanced if we can find some way to assert our sense of control. That process itself is modified by such things as our age and the state of our health, which often lead us to rely on others (our physician, our spouse). When different samples of illness categories, different samples of patients, different researchers with different questions all converge on highly similar results, then we can feel greater confidence in our understanding of the processes involved.

Externally-Caused Undesirable Events as Instances of Deliberate Threat to Our Control

In the case of events which truly are accidental, we are left with the term "bad luck" to explain how that undesirable event was "caused." But sometimes our stressful events come not from the vague term "bad luck" but from obvious sources such as other people or the ways that our environment is arranged against us at the time. Being put in prison, for instance, may be "bad luck," but a more rational analysis would place the cause in the perpetrator's initial unlawful conduct, and then in the externally-controlling behavior of police, the courts, and the law and, ultimately, the prison administrators. You do not need the term "bad luck" to explain incarceration, at least in a just society.

Given this class of experiences, I can now discuss our second category of externally-caused undesirable events: The negative events which arise from deliberate, intentional actions against the person. There are many such events in our life in spite of our attempts to avoid them. The initial research on this class of undesirable events was focused on a type of experience that is unfortunately all too-common: Rape.

Rape is in fact no accident. It is a deliberately-executed assault on another person. It is inflicted by the perpetrator on an unwilling victim, and it is a crime in the eyes of society. But it takes on specific properties if viewed from the viewpoint of control theory. We know from the research of Janoff-Bulman and Wortman on paraplegics and quadriplegics that to assert control over an accident at least can show the benefits of believing in one's control over the event. But in the case of rape, it is not chance or bad luck that it the most obvious cause: It is overwhelmingly a male-initiated sexual assault as a conscious act of asserting control over a woman. Even at that, though, there may be some extenuating circumstances in which the "ultimate, true" cause of the event may be ambiguous about the woman's role. But certainly from an event-causation perspective it could not have occurred without the active control by the male. That is a matter for the police and the courts to decide, but personal control research provides valuable insights into how to understand the victim's reaction to the experience.

Ronnie Janoff-Bulman[6] (again) pioneered the research in the psychological reactions of women to such an awful experience. Previous psychological research on depression had suggested to her that if people blame themselves for bad experiences, that blaming can be a major factor in leading them to have depressive symptoms. This may sound counter to her other research findings on accident victims, but she had the impressive insight that there were different ways to blame oneself. In fact, the very concept of "blame" itself needed to be investigated. One can blame one's *personality,* one's character, or one can blame one's *behavior,* one's actions, the things that the person did. These are very different entities. The question is, does this distinction make a difference, and in this case, a difference to women who have experienced rape?

To study this, she sought professional opinions from the administrators and staff of 38 women's rape crisis centers from around the country. She sent them a survey questionnaire to get data on the types of causal explanations that their clients expressed. She asked them to report what percentage of their clients expressed what she was calling "characterological self-blame" and how many were expressing what she called "behavioral self-blame."

Here are examples from the category of characterological self-blame:

That's the kind of person I am.
I'm too trusting.
I misjudge people all the time.
I'm so stupid, I deserved it.
I'm weak, I can't say No.

Here are examples from the other category, behavioral selfblame:

I shouldn't have ignored him.
I should have locked my windows.
I shouldn't have been hitchhiking.
I shouldn't have been in that alley.

Janoff-Bulman found that 60% of the respondents were making behavioral self-blame, whereas 19% were making characterological self-blame. The other participant reports were mixtures and not clearly either of these two categories. From a control and personal mastery perspective, these are very different categories of perceived causes. Note that both categories are blaming of the self; there is no very clear hint of blaming the male involved in the incident. But blaming one's behavior is indeed a much more controllable cause: The message is something like, "Next time, I will be alert and I won't let it happen to me again." But if one is blaming one's core, basic self, one's character by thinking such a thought as, "That's the kind of person I am," then that is a much more difficult path to change; how does one change one's very character? Janoff-Bulman discussed specifically how blaming one's *behavior* reflects a control-maintenance orientation, and it suggests that the woman should be focused on future avoidability of such an incident ever happening again.

Dr. Patricia Frazer followed this study with a more intensive investigation of the types of causes rape victims make about their experience.[7] She developed an multi-item questionnaire about possible causes and then administered it to a sample of 67 women who were in treatment for rape in a hospital-based treatment facility (as opposed to the therapeutic staff surveyed by Janoff-Bulman). In her study, she basically asked each woman to indicate how much she blamed her behavior and how much she blamed her character traits for the experience. She found that most of the patients did not clearly distinguish sharply between the two categories.

It turns out that with a more intensive analysis with deeply-probing items that it is difficult to blame one's behavior without in some way also implicating one's character. But fortunately other questions on the survey revealed that the patients thought that they could not have avoided the experience just as we saw in the accidents' study of Janoff-Bulman and Wortman but they felt that could avoid the experience *in the future*. Both of these kinds of responses were most clearly related to their patients' improvement and adjustment after the experience.

Frazier found that some of her respondents were showing high levels of depression after their experience, while others were better off. The difference between them, as you might expect, has to do with how they thought about the past and the future and how their own personal control could be engaged in their future lives. Those who thought that they had shown poor judgment and that that they were the "victim type" were more depressed than those who thought that they could take control of their future by being more alert, more careful, and more in control of their situational events.

So when we combine the results of the Janoff-Bulman and Wortman study with Frazier's, we can sketch a fuller picture of how beliefs in one's mastery play a major role in enhancing good adjustment to traumatic experiences. The study of the spinal cord injury patents led us to conclude that their believing that they themselves were the cause of the problem was helpful for adjustment. But Frazier's results modify that: It is more than just seeing the self as the cause. If you believe that you cannot control your future, as one who cannot take care of yourself and manage the events of your life, then that is a recipe for poor adjustment. It is when you see things as *changeable*, as thinking that you can control the future, that you can change things to avoid negative experiences, that you are most likely to experience a better, healthier recovery.

In fact, Frazier suggests a major shift of focus in our therapies: Not to encourage clients to blame themselves for undesirable events, but to focus on *changeable* parts of their lives and take action on them. And of course, this means to focus your control efforts on changeable things, not blaming locked-in character traits. From our personal control perspective, if things are changeable, they are personally controllable. In retrospect, it seems as if Jeff Lewis clearly thought that his life circumstances were changeable, and he did that by contacting prosthetics manufacturers to give him equipment that he could use to change his life, which he did to an impressive degree.

External Loss of Control in Institutional Environments
You will recall from my discussion in Chapter 3 of the work of Frederick Herzberg on worker motivation in organizations

and business environments. His distinction between "hygiene factors" and "motivator factors" showed the distinctly different effects when managements focus on factors external to the worker such as changing work place conditions without consideration of psychological factors such as a desire for a sense of successful achievement and personal growth. Of course, from what we now have learned from more recent research, I would add personal mastery beliefs and personal control to the side of motivator factors. Following his insights, we need to search through the work setting to find perhaps hidden and subtle ways in which changing environmental conditions can work against our workers having a greater sense of personal mastery.

You may have noticed that the majority of the studies on loss of control were conducted in institutional settings such as hospitals and rape treatment facilities. These institutions are founded on the principle of helping someone in need, either physical or psychological. There is no question that these organizations are helpful in many ways and certainly they are needed as a societal response to people in distress. But the word "helpful" means different things in different contexts. In reading this book, you are by now well-acquainted with the need to be specific about what is involved in "help," since it implies that an external cause of an event or set of events is being applied to the individual person in a condition of dependency on others. In this sense, "help" is a signal to the person that their own personal mastery of their environment is not functioning well enough for them to be independent; as a consequence, they are at least temporarily "in need," and society has come along to provide that needed help. Are we always sure that such help is indeed useful? Is there a danger that when we help someone we are potentially undermining their sense of personal mastery?

I will show in the next chapter that, in fact, there is a process called "undermining," in which an external event (in this case a positive event) actually reduces the person's own motivation for controlling their environment. At any rate, it is a serious question to pose: How much is helping a threat to one's sense of personal control? How well do people do when they are put into a situation in which control over their daily living is deliberately placed in their environment rather than inside them?

This is exactly what happens when we place our elderly in nursing homes and extended care facilities. Society has made these institutional settings available to care for the elderly who are judged as no longer capable of high levels of their own self-care. In our language here, these are places where control over the welfare of the person is handled by the staff. As such, they would be considered as controlling environments, but environments of external rather than internal control. Thinking of them this way automatically raises the Person/Environment (PXE) congruence approach which I discussed in Chapter 1. In this case, this would involve an investigation of how people rated their opportunities for control over the events of their daily living compared to what control is actually available to them.

Barbara Felton and Eva Kahana[8] in fact investigated this issue by studying a sample of 124 residents of three different homes for the aged in Michigan. Residents were interviewed about their control beliefs concerning how much they felt that they could do something about their daily lives such as maintaining their privacy and their activity and engagement in the residence's activities. Responses were scored on the dimension of internal/external control (as assessed by the sample test I presented in Chapter 2), control asserted either by themselves or by other people such as the staff, their family, friends or other people. The investigators also assessed the residents' adjustment to the home, their morale, and their satisfaction with their lives, and the home staff also provided ratings of how well they thought the residents were doing.

The results were quite consistent with our control and mastery perspective. On the great majority of the measures, both self-rated and staff-rated, the residents who had higher *externality* beliefs were better off than those who had higher internality beliefs! Although much of what I have said so far would seem to argue that externality is related to poorer outcomes, believing that staff and other people were more responsible for control over their lives was helpful to those who had beliefs in external control. Stated the other way, those who held higher internal beliefs *in this particular setting* were not doing as well. Felton and Kahana argued that this shows the power of following a PXE model in studying well-being in people. High internal beliefs in one's personal mastery and control are not always going to be related to better adjustment. It depends on the environment.

This finding takes on special meaning in the light of a lengthy series of studies on nursing home environments conducted by Margaret Baltes and her colleagues (summarized in Baltes and Reisenzein).[9] These investigators had their research staff actually observe resident-staff patterns of interactions during the course of daily observation sessions. The specific focus of their study was on what occurred as the resident engaged in daily behaviors and how the staff reacted to those behaviors. Across a number of observation sessions, they found that when the residents relied upon the staff, when they manifested *dependency-type* behaviors, the members of the staff were highly responsive, supportive and helpful. However, when the residents acted independently and were not reliant on the staff, the staff was unresponsive and in fact tended to ignore the resident! The results indicated that highcontrol environments such as nursing homes encourage dependence and external control; actions of self-control and independence receive little or no feedback. A quote from the investigators is instructive:

...we find a consistently and immediately supportive social environment for dependent self-care behavior, whereas independent self-care behaviors are rarely followed by observable responses from the social environment.

If residence staff does not reward independence-type behaviors, then those behaviors will tend to fade and drop out of the person's responses to their environment. A personal mastery perspective would argue that rewarding independence-type responses would be related to more healthful outcomes for the person.

Stephen Wolk[10] has reported that mental health and general well-being of residents are directly related to the constraining or open-living nature of residential facilities. He studied personal control in older adults in two different types of retirement living: (1) a retirement village stressing high individual control where they own their own homes, provide for their own needs, and in other ways have a lifestyle of high personal responsibility, (2) a more traditional nursing home setting, where the residents' needs were met by organized and structured staff procedures, the rules are clearly defined and a set daily schedule is followed, with only occasional allowance for more personal choices. These retirees responded to the Rotter Locus of Control scale (described in Chapter 2) and a set of scales assessing, among other things, the residents' sense of satisfaction with their living, adjustment to their settings, and their activity level. Of course, both groups of residents contained people who scored high or low on the personal control scales, giving us comparisons within each type of setting for both types of residents.

The results of this study showed significant effects from a PXE fit approach. The high internal residents reported higher life satisfaction, better adjustment and higher levels of activity in the more open and free setting of the retirement village, but none of these relationships held for the lower personal control setting of the residential facility. This shows that the environment can foster internality and better adjustment if it is unstructured and open, giving the high internality person more freedom for growth and adjustment, rather than imposing structure and relatively less freedom. This conclusion was supported by another study[11] where internals were shown to get more benefits from an unstructured therapy, and externals showed more improvement from directive, structured therapy.

Learned Helplessness

There is an underlying theme in these studies: How does putting control outside of the person and in the environment develop longer-term consequences for control perceptions and actions? When elderly people are moved into retirement and assisted-care facilities, there has already been a loss of personal control, at least to a degree significant enough to make that decision necessary. Clearly we would not want to put someone in that type of situation if there were not a need to do so. But that leaves a big question unexplored: What effects do such environments have on control beliefs and actions separately from the debilitating effects of advanced age or serious illness or, in the case of prisons, prior antisocial behavior? A sample of research participants without significant pre-existing control limitations is needed to get a true measure of the effects of being exposed to a controlling environment.

A landmark series of experimental studies, arising initially in the animal learning research tradition, showed great promise and then those studies were applied to human psychology research. You will no doubt recall the early studies on animal learning by the Russian physiologist Ivan Pavlov, in which he studied how animals (dogs, in this case) could learn to respond to a buzzer sound. He found that for learning to occur there had to be a previous period in which the buzzer was paired with a bit of food. Ordinarily a dog would salivate to the food independent of any other conditions, but Pavlov was able to condition the animals to salivate to a buzzer presented just immediately before the presentation of the food. By conditioning, the buzzer took on the ability to elicit the salivation as the food had. This classical conditioning process explains a number of learning phenomena, and now is considered one of the standard models of how learning occurs.

In a pioneering series of research studies extending this model of learning, Martin Seligman and Steven Maier[12] argued that a key to this phenomenon is the nature of the uncontrollable environmental conditions. The dog had no control over the buzzer or over receiving the food. But Seligman and Maier wondered if the animal's learning experiences *prior to* the final buzzer/response/food connection was made would be a significant influence on the dog's subsequent behavior. In effect, they wanted to build in a prior learning history but in this case one of complete uncontrollability. Basically, the question was, will an animal be able to learn the response/reward connection if it earlier had learned that its responses have no effective control over its environment?

The methodology to conduct this type of experiment is rather complicated and I will highlight only the most helpful details. Briefly, the main technique was to put a restraining harness on the dog before actually beginning the training condition, then give a signal followed by a harmless but upsetting mild shock to the animal. Since it is restrained, the animal cannot jump away from the shock; it has to experience that uncontrollable noxious stimulus several times over a set of learning sessions. This situation signals to the animal that it has lost behavioral control over its environment. Then, after that experience, the animal is put into a learning box where, if the dog makes a simple jump over a low hurdle, it can avoid the mild shock which will follow after the buzzer. That is an example of a "learned avoidance" response. The key response for the dog is to learn the connection between jumping over the low hurdle and thus avoiding the shock, something any dog under normal circumstances can learn easily. The dog has its own version of control motivation which it can easily exercise when given an easy escape response to learn.

To their amazement, the research team found that dogs which had the pre-training in the uncontrollable condition (the harness condition) would not make any attempts to jump over the hurdle to escape the threat from the buzzer and the correlated shock. After the buzzer sounded, the animal could have jumped over the hurdle and would not have experienced the tingling from the shock. In fact, a control group of naïve animals who had not been harnessed and exposed to the prior buzzer/shock experience learned quickly to make the small jump and easily avoided getting any shock. But the dogs with the prior conditioning history of having to being exposed to the buzzer/shock combination without being able to control it or to avoid it (because of the harness restraint) did not even try to avoid the shock by making the simple response of jumping over the hurdle. The dogs simply sat down after the buzzer sounded and underwent the unpleasant tingling. Time and time again, they made no effort to avoid the shock after the buzzer sounded. They never really started getting active again in the experimental situation, and so had to experience the unpleasant shocks.

Seligman and his team found that they had trained in a response of helplessness in their experimental animals compared to the control animals. They called this *"learned helplessness,"* a perfectly descriptive term for exactly what they were observing; the dogs exposed to an environment of uncontrollable experience had lost any sense of making a controlling response. What this helplessness response looks like is a "giving up;" in our language in this book, it is in fact a failure to make a personal control response. The dog *could not* in fact make a controlling response in the initial training sessions, but in the second session it *would not* make a controlling response.

To an observer who might look at the animal in the second phase without knowing what had happened in the first phase, the animals looked depressed. They were passive, withdrawn, unresponsive, quiet, retreated inwardly. If you saw a human being in that state, you would call that person "depressed." After these initial studies, many investigators and clinical practitioners now have come to think of living in an environment of uncontrollable events as a model of how people become depressed. The question explores the way that humans give up on controlling their world, a key symptom of depression.

In fact, a direct test of the learned helplessness effect and control beliefs in humans was developed by Donald Hiroto.[13] He developed a two-phase experiment in which the first session involved exposure to an uncontrollable irritating stimulus (a fairly loud 110 decibels tone, rather than a shock) which the participants could stop from occurring in an "escapable" condition or they could not stop, an "inescapable" condition. Then they were moved to an apparatus with a lever which they could twist to the left or to the right. They were given the belief that they could stop the tone if they could figure out which way to move the lever; the lever either would prevent the tone from occurring in the first place or, if it had gone off, they could escape it if they could figure out the correct moves of the lever. The experimenter kept track of the speed with which they made their controlling attempts.

A particularly interesting feature of this experiment from our personal control approach is that, before the experiment actually began, the participants answered a pencil-and-paper questionnaire assessing their beliefs in internal or external control (as I described in Chapter 2). So in this study the effects of prior personality trait beliefs in control were crossed with a method which first prevented them or allowed them to have actual control over the aversive tone. Again, here we have a test of the PXE approach to personal control.

The data were quite clear. First, participants exposed to the inescapable initial condition showed poorer response in the second phase, the standard learned helplessness outcome. But trait personal mastery influenced this process: The high internal belief in personal control participants were *faster* in both avoiding the tone and escaping from it if it had already occurred than the externals. As you might expect, the external participants, demonstrating more learned helplessness, took a greater number of trials to learn how to avoid the tone than the internals. Interpreting this find from a personal control mastery, they already live in a world where they believe that they do not have much control.

A raft of similar studies has confirmed these basic findings. A quote from Hiroto sums up this literature:

In conclusion, this study demonstrated that helplessness can be experimentally induced in man wholly parallel to helplessness in animals (p.192).

Personal Control Can Be Merely Perceived, Not Actual

Learned helplessness conditions seem widely prevalent in society; it is often difficult to get a sense of personal control over many of our daily experiences. Having a personality disposition such as being an internal on a locus of control test or a personal mastery test enhances our adjustment capacity, but inevitably we do sometimes confront uncontrollable situations. But this raises the question of whether or not controlling actions have to be actually engaged, carried out to completion, of if just having a *belief* in control without actually performing it is sufficient to sustain our well-being? Is it possible to separate out actual control from the internal perception of control, as several of our PXE studies suggested, but is actually doing the behavior to control the situation necessary for us to cope well with the situation? Remember that the standard pencil-and-paper questionnaires assessing personal control target control beliefs; they do not typically list actual controlling behaviors that the person may or may not have manifested in various situations in their life.

In the pioneering research of David Glass, Jerome Singer and Lucy Friedman, this question was directly confronted. In their book, *Urban Stress*[14] they argued that most of us are living in modern environments filled with uncontrollable experiences, and the stress of those experiences can have serious psychological and health effects (the title of their book, *Urban Stress,* suggests the scope of their focus). The question was, can control beliefs be separated from control behaviors, and the effects of each assessed independently?

To test their general model of stress, in cooperation with Lucy Singer, they developed a laboratory analogue of stressful urban environment.[15] They conducted a two-phase experiment in which respondents were first exposed to uncontrollable stressful experiences, in this case a randomly-spaced loud blast of noise behind them as they worked on complicated cognitive tasks. Such tasks were chosen to detect any harmful effects resulting from the noise on performance. Knowing the ability of people to adjust to their environment, even a stressful environment, the investigators predicted that the respondents would be able to adjust to the noise and, compared to a control group which did not receive the uncontrollable noise, the respondents would perform at about the same level. In fact that is what they found: Successful adjustment and competent performance was found in those participants subjected to the unpleasant uncontrollable noise, and not significantly worse than control participants not experiencing that noise.

But the investigators had a different aim in this study, as reflected in the second phase of their experimental conditions. Their intent was to study the *cost* of adaptation. Yes, in fact we can adjust to uncontrollability and stressful experiences, but we do so by a steady wearing-down of our resilience resources at a serious cost later on. This exhaustion of resources should be especially obvious if we are faced with even more, out-of-control stressful events. It was in the second, post-stress phase of their study that they expected the wearing down of the stress induced by the noise to finally appear in the performance of their respondents. The experiment was actually a study in what psychologists call "frustration tolerance."

The key to the entire experiment was a subtle but important difference. Just before the respondents has actually started working on their Phase 1 problem solving tasks, one-half of them, those assigned to the "button condition" were shown a microswitch attached to one side of their chair. They were told that, if they wanted to, they could press the switch and it would terminate the noise for the remainder of the experiment. The other half of the respondents did not have a button and of course they did not receive any information about the switch (the "no button" condition). In effect, the button group had control available to them should they feel it necessary to use it; the comparison group participants had no such control available to them.

In this second phase of the experiment, all of the respondents were given an extensive set of behavioral endurance stress tests to determine just how well they could keep on performing, but now without the noise being presented. This test of endurance and failure to perform was the key measure. The results in this second phase showed a big difference: The "button group" continued working on their tasks about 4 times as much as the "no button" group: this comparison group gave up very quickly and terminated the experiment whereas the "button" group kept going on.

This large and dramatic difference clearly showed that having a way to control a situation provided the respondents with superior stress-tolerance ability that led them to work harder and more consistently even when the world was frustrating. Stated another way, having no (perceived) control over a stressful, unpleasant experience can lead you, later on, to lack the ability to deal well with tasks requiring a significant level of cognitive, problem-solving ability.

And now comes the most intriguing finding of this study. No one person in the "button" condition ever actually pressed the button. None, not one! They went through the first-phase stressful experiences just the same as the "no button" participants. In that sense, all participants had exactly the same first-phase experience, yet the "button" group showed superior frustration tolerance *later on*. That can only mean that the high control instructions had a purely mental effect: No controlling behaviors were actually needed to provide the "button" participants with perceived control. Mastery is in the mind and need not be actually exercised to have positive effects, even in stressful circumstances such as the frustrating, high-stress situation presented in this task.

In Sum

Overall, the unique body of studies I discussed in this chapter represents a creative and useful melding of personal mastery and control theory with obvious clinical relevance when people are forced to deal with undesirable events in their lives. We now know that personal control can have both positive and negative consequences for a person's well-being, depending on the freedom offered to the person by the environment. But this chapter has had a slant to it: The consequences are negative for the person when the events in the environment are stressful, undesirable, or harmful and there is a blocking or hindrance to exercising personal freedom of action. Sometimes that has positive benefits; for instance, when the person's health is poor and dependency on the environment can be helpful in sustaining well-being. Personal control can be supplanted by acceptance and yielding when the environment actually is uncontrollable, at least by oneself. We have a range of adaptation capacities of which direct personal control is only one device.

Our resilience in the face of unyielding environmental events is only one step in human adaptation and resilience. The "button-no button" study is a marvelous example of the power of personal mastery beliefs. The results suggest that confidence, a sense of competence and adaptability, and such beliefs can sustain us through nearly anything the world can put in front of us.

Now the question arises, what about *desirable* events. How do we fare when we are in an environment that allows us to pursue our own personal forms of control compared to environments that in fact provide us with positive events outside of our own control? This set of questions exactly mirrors what I have presented in this chapter. So now, in the next chapter, let us explore the world of things we like, such as events and how they relate to our personal causation.

Chapter 5

Desirable Events Support Our Mastery

In this chapter I want to turn our attention to the desirable events in our lives. For most of us, and perhaps naturally, it is a main goal of life to have as many positive experiences as we can. While that may seem natural, I do not want you to be too hasty or too casual about that goal: Caution is advised and, as I did in the Introduction, I am again raising the issue for you to consider. There are hidden threats to our sense of personal mastery in that pursuit and you should not assume that achieving desirable events will automatically be to your long-term benefit. While this caution may strike you as misdirected, the logic of the personal mastery model leads to it as a distinct possibility.

In many ways, this pursuit of the desirable is "where the action is." Surveys and experimental research has shown that people report having many more desirable events in their lives than undesirable ones, in some cases by a factor of 2 or 3 times as many.[1] Since desirable events are more under our personal control than undesirable ones, then this suggests that people should be free to exercise their personal mastery and have the opportunity to create lives of virtually unlimited happiness.

If we were to attempt this lofty goal, I suggest that the consideration should be based on personal control theory and data rather than simple, shoot-from-the-hip wishful thinking. Given what we know of the many benefits of desirable events, one could propose, seriously, that we should try to create an ideal society where everyone would experience undeviatingly positive experiences. What a life! But anyone thinking about proposing a serious public policy along these lines should be informed by the remarkable thinking of Philip Brickman and

Donald Campbell.[2] Of course, we should always strive to base any public policy on the best knowledge we have, and a lot of research has shown us the broad-ranging effects that positive events have for our physical and mental health. The idea of trying to create and implement that policy certainly should get serious consideration. Ignoring for a moment how it would be done, the core idea is how to provide a continuous stream of positive experiences for people. Indeed, why would *not* that be an ideal society?

Brickman and Campbell argue, again logically, that such a course would be doomed to failure. Even if it could somehow be brought about, you would inevitably be creating for yourself what they call a "hedonic treadmill." It would be a treadmill because of the inherent operation of what psychologists call the formation and functioning of *adaptation level* processing. This model of perceptual processes, pioneered by Harry Helson,[3] posits that our judgments of the world are shaped by the totality of our prior experiences. Helson has developed a mathematical formula that basically averages all of one's prior experience into a single point, a point of reference against which all new events are judged. For example, if someone has grown up in Fairbanks, Alaska, a temperature of 50 degrees Fahrenheit would find them barefoot and basking in shorts. But someone who has grown up in Yuma, Arizona, would consider 50 degrees so cold that it would require warm clothes and heavy socks. What is the difference? The Fairbanks native has grown up with a mean daily temperature of 26.9 (most recent statistics) so 50 degrees is detectably hotter than that. The Yuma resident growing up with an average daily temperature of 74.2 (most recent value) would call that same objectively measured 50 degrees pretty chilly. In Helson's mathematical model of human perception processes, the average of one's past experiences is actually a point of adaptation, an adaptation level (AL). This AL sets our judgment standards for perceiving our world, in this case our world of heat and cold. The AL itself is a neutral point which carries no particular feelings of pleasant or unpleasant. It is our comparison point, our standard for judging events: Those events registered as above it (in our examples) are judged as plusses and desirable, and those below it register as minuses, undesirable. Any value at exactly that point, or very near it, would not register as either warm or cold; it would have a neutral value and we would not feel one way or the other about it.

Now Brickman and Campbell argue that attempting to create a society of undeviatingly positive experiences is doomed to failure. Any new positive experience will be melded into one's prior AL and will itself become neutral as a result of it becoming part of the new average. A short-term feeling of positivity will get quickly lost into the neutral point of average. To solve that problem, one would have to arrange for more positive experiences for the person, detectably more positive than the neutral point. But these new experiences, in turn would meld into the average, so more and more and more positive experiences would have to be engineered for the person to keep feeling positively. But again they will become neutral by being averaged into the AL. Brickman and Campbell call this "a hedonic treadmill," an endless need for more and more positive events to beat the blahs, the feeling of neutrality. Undeviatingly positive experiences, seemingly an ideal society, can never be successful; the averaging is inexorable.

While this entire discussion is of course purely theoretical, the science on which it is based is both valid and reliable. It gives us pause to think about our own personal lives: Would you want to find yourself in an endless quest for more and more positive experiences only to find out that it is not working? Should you pursue positive experiences endlessly in the hope of feeling better and better and better? Of course, it turns out in real life that we have plenty of negative and neutral experiences that reduce the neutral point. The real diversity of events has the result that we can actually feel good about even mildly positive experiences. Life itself is filled with all sorts of events, not just one type, fortunately. Still, though, many of us spend much of our life searching out changes for more and more positive experiences.

But while the theory of adaptation level processes is sound, my colleague Alex Zautra and I thought that the logic was based on a potentially faulty model of what was being called "positive events." The fault lay in assuming that all positive events were identical in terms of their positivity and how they got it. I am sure that you can see where I am going with this. We argued that some events that are positive are the result of the actions of the individual while other events are positive but arise outside of the control of the individual. The role of personal mastery and event causation had been ignored in the controversy about how to build a better society: "Better" in what terms? we asked. If I ask you what you think about the first letter grade of A you got in school, I suspect that you still feel pretty good about it. You are not going to feel neutral about "an outstanding personal achievement" in your life, to give you one of our questionnaire items to test this model. On the other hand, to get "A reduction in course requirements" from your teacher (also from our list of events) is a positive event but one not under your control. You may have forgotten about it by now. You would no doubt find it desirable if your boss told you that you would be given a lighter workload because of your excellent past performance.

With these ideas and personal mastery theory to guide us, we conducted a study of personal causation and the hedonic treadmill. We wanted to pit the effects of desirable and undesirable events against the causes of those events, internal and external. I discussed some of the results of that study in Chapter 3.[4] In it, we labeled self-created positive events "Positive Origin" events, and positive events arising from outside of us, from external causes, we called "Positive Pawn" events. Here we were applying the origin-pawn thinking of Richard deCharms.[5] To reiterate some of the points I made about that study, we showed that experiencing a higher number of positive origin events was related to higher quality of life reports, but higher experiencing of positive *pawn* events was related to participants' reports of poorer quality of life. There was no evidence that the externally-caused positive events were related to greater happiness or an improved quality of life. The experience of being a pawn, a passive recipient even of positive events, is not a good outcome for people; pawnness swamped event positivity.

The implications of what the data are telling us are important to consider. We all seek positive events in our lives, but there is a mixed message here: Pursuing positive events over which we have no control, such as gambling, scratch lottery tickets, and hoping for a wealthy relative to give us money, are not wise paths to take. I shall discuss these blind alleys in this chapter. Perhaps Brickman and Campbell's model of the hedonic treadmill is too limited in its applicability. The key is not necessarily the positive event, *per se*, but the event that we ourselves create and thereby gain from the exercise of our personal mastery that gives events their favorable effects on us. Perhaps if we could engineer a society in which people are able to exercise their personal control to obtain positive events which they achieve through their own self-causation, then maybe we can create "the good society." I am arguing theoretically, of course, but the data confirm the basic outlines of this possibility.

The Key to Our Well-Being is the Choices We Make

A key issue I have not yet discussed is a seemingly simple one: How does belief in our own personal mastery become activated so that we can pursue our positive events and avoid negative ones? What is it that weaves our beliefs into an action pattern for actually engaging with the desirable opportunities and undesirable stresses in our environments?

There are many ways one could approach these questions, but the research I have been presenting here suggests that the most fruitful way to approach it would be through the concept of *choice* or, in our terms, *personal choice*. To get a good definition of this concept, I entered the word "choice" in a Google search and got back 1,580,000,000 links. Narrowing my search with the word "free choice," I got 120,000,000 hits, and "personal choice" returned 59,300,000. There is obviously a lot to say about choice.

An insightful treatment of the concept recently has been suggested by Sheena Iyengar in her book, *The Art of Choice* (2010).[6] Her definition is:

When we speak of choice, what we mean is the ability to exercise control over ourselves and our environment... The ability to choose well is arguably the most powerful tool for controlling our environment. (pp. 6-7).

This definition explicitly points to the role of choice over our own actions and over the environment. Our treatment of both major and small events has been based on results of studies in which the person either had choices over courses of action, or did not. Of course, for the big things such as choosing a career, choosing to get married, choosing to retire, then the paths we choose are major decisions that take a lot of our time and energy; they are exercises of our sense of personal mastery and we are fully conscious of how much we need to be able to control as many aspects of the choice as possible. This holds true for both desirable and undesirable events. Once that choice is made, our entire lifestyle gets changed and redirected; our deliberate choices can have a huge impact on us.

But these major events are relatively rare in our lives, as important as they are. In Chapter 3, I discussed the tight linkage between event causation and event valuation. The more mundane events which Alex Zautra and I call "demands and desires" and Richard Lazarus and Alan Kanner and their colleagues call "hassles and uplifts" are equally significant to our well-being because, fundamentally they involve choices. Now you would ordinarily think of something like taking a big vacation would be more significant to your well-being as, for instance, choosing to wear a blue shirt rather than a white one. But logically and psychologically speaking, they are both exercises of our personal choices and in that sense they are *psychologically* equal. Imagine being told that you cannot choose what to wear, or that you cannot go outside of your house for 24 hours. That would be distressing indeed, not because your house is not pleasant, but because you are not allowed to choose what to do with your time for 24 hours. So, in overview, the key to exercising our personal mastery is the active act of choosing a preferred way of responding.

When Playing Isn't Playing Anymore

We make choices to maximize our gains and to minimize our losses, to achieve desirable outcomes and to avoid undesirable ones. When we freely choose a course of action, we usually do so in the expectation that it will pay off in one of these two ways, or both. Our expectancy is a fundamental component of choosing a particular course of action. But what if the choice leads to an unexpected consequence? We freely made a choice and that exercise of our personal mastery gives the action positive value. But the *consequences* of a choice have value as well, and in many cases those consequences actually degrade our sense of control. This issue of how expectancy and choice relate to each other is a major key to our success in dealing with the events of our lives.

A systematic approach to disentangle these components of our personal mastery was developed by a series of carefully controlled laboratory studies on children's choices to do "fun" things by Mark Lepper, David Green, and Richard Nisbett[7] and many later investigators. Their famous "Magic Markers" study went to the heart of choices, motivations, and the consequences of our choices.

To demonstrate the importance of a freely-chosen action, the investigators chose children in their Stanford University childcare school as participants, giving them an opportunity to play with Magic Markers, a pen-like device for drawing and marking. Needless to say, this interesting activity would not require any special inducement to get the children to play. Such motivation to play is called "intrinsic motivation" where the personal cause of the playing is internal to the child, as opposed to some form of external inducement to get them to perform the behavior. But the role of the inducement might actually have damaging effects on an event's positive value.

They examined this possibility in a two-phase experiment: An initial phase in which children were given the Magic Marker/drawing pad materials to play with freely and a follow-up session to play again 1-2 weeks later. Unknown to the children, they had been randomly assigned to one of three experimental conditions that were nested within the first phase of the experiment: (1) Expected Reward, (2) Unexpected Reward, and a (3) No Instructions condition.

In the Expected Reward condition, the child was given the following instructions:

...there's a man (lady) who's come to the nursery school for a few days to see what kinds of pictures boys and girls like to draw with magic markers. Would you like to draw some picture for him (her)? (there was a pause, and all children said "Yes"). *And he's brought along a few of these Good Player Awards to give to boys and girls who will help him out by drawing some pictures for him(her). See? It's got a big gold*

star and a bright red ribbon, and there's a place here for your name and your school. Would you like to win one of these Good Player Awards?

Of course all of the children in this experimental condition said "Yes" and they did play with the Magic Markers, drawing whatever pictures that they wanted (freely chose) to draw. And then, with much fanfare, the child's name was written onto the Award Certificate and then put up on the bulletin board, receiving public notice as a Good Player.

Another set of the nursery school children were randomly assigned to the "Unexpected Award" condition. They were given almost exactly the same speech except the timing was different. Here the children were asked if they wanted to draw some pictures and, when they (all) said "Yes," they were simply given their Magic Marker and a pad of paper to draw their pictures; no mention was made of an award. However, *after* they had played with their materials, the children were given exactly the same treatment: The same speech (slightly reworded), and their names written on the Gold Star Award certificates which were then posted on the bulletin board along with the other Good Players in the school. Note that the two groups received nearly identical treatment instructions except that the first group agreed to play with the materials *in order to get the award* while the second group got the award *after* they had made the personal decision to play. The distinction here is important to note and it centers around the *timing* and location of the cause of the reward. The first group's decision was intrinsically motivated and not under the control of the externally-announced award because the children had not been told about it. But for the second group the reward was clearly announced prior to the opportunity to play and it acted as an external cause to the children in making their decision to play or not to play.

The third group of children, the comparison group who were also randomly assigned to their condition, never heard anything about any award or any Magic Marker play opportunities. They simply kept playing as usual on the school playground while the other groups were engaging in their drawing activities.

One to two weeks' later, all of the children were taken to the Magic Marker play room and left alone for a "free play" period. No award was mentioned this time and the children were totally on their own to do whatever they wanted. Whatever playing they did this time would be based only on their personal choice and motivation. During this period of exposure to the drawing materials, the children were carefully timed by an experimenter behind a one-way mirror observing them and timing/assessing how much of their free-play time was actually spent in drawing. This is a direct quantitative measure of intrinsic motivation: The investigators could now determine how much time the children spent actually drawing as opposed to doing something else in that room. Also, cleverly, the experimenters kept and stored the children's drawings so that the quality of the children's play could be scored by trained art judges, scoring for quality of artistic effort being reflected in the drawings. The children assigned to the comparison group who had heard nothing about awards or the drawing activity were also given the chance to draw and the time they spent doing so was recorded and their drawings were retained for later scoring on quality.

The results of the study were quite clear. In the second, free-play session, those children who were in the Unexpected Award group played significantly *more* with the Magic Markers than the Expected Award group, and the quality of their drawings was judged as significantly poorer than the Unexpected Award group. The comparison group children played about the same amount as the Expected reward group, and the quality of their drawings also was scored as relatively poor also. The group that stood out in terms of less dedication to the drawing task, and the quality of their performance, was the group that performed the playing with the reward as their initial motivation. Those who had freely chosen to play performed in a superior manner.

Interpreting their results, Lepper, Green and Nisbett suggested that the presence of the Award *undermined* the children's otherwise intrinsic motivation to play with the Magic Markers. Those children who earlier had played with the fun game *because* they wanted to get an award ended up playing less, and doing poorer quality work, than all of the other children in the study. The Unexpected Award children were presented with an opportunity to play simply because they could choose to do so, or not; they were the causal agents of their own activity, and only later did they even find out about the Good Player award. It was their own action, not someone else's and not some external "pay" that induced them to play in the first place. So the results showed that Expected Award condition had in effect "bought off" the children by promising them an award *if* they would play. In turn, in the second phase, when no reward was mentioned, their motivation to play had been undermined; they showed less time on task and poorer motivation to do a good job.

The implications of this study, and the dozens of others that followed up on it, are profound not only for our school children but for our entire social system of inducements for performance. School could be a wonderful experience, a wonderland of toys and books and friends, with children engaged in pursing interesting and stimulating alternatives. But from childhood on, society gives grades and awards to children in school, and those children learn to work and study in order to get those grades and gold stars. But by the very arrangements of the school's environment, they are put into a situation where they end up not motivated to learn for the sake of learning, they learn for the sake of getting the external rewards. If those reward symbols go away (no reward was mentioned in the second phase of the experiment), so does the motivation for performing. You can conclude that to keep the undermined children engaged in the play activity, the external rewards would have to be maintained forever. That course of action seems likely to fail because it might get us back to Helson's adaptation level (AL) problem, putting us on an endless "hedonic reward treadmill." Making performance contingent on a reward removes motivation for doing the performance for the joy and fun of just doing it. Pay or awards or grades are forms of external pressure, and they do not get the motivation moved internally where it would endure as a lasting cause of the behavior.

This study shows how play can become work... through pay, timed to occur before the person gets a meaningful personal choice, the play is in effect already coerced behavior before it can be freely chosen. Once the play behavior gets attached to pay, then there is an undermining of the original intrinsic motivation and it declines if not disappears altogether.

I can relay a story to you that you will find interesting from the perspective of undermining phenomena. There is a publically available story going around that I find neatly encapsulates it. I have tried to track down the original source for a real-world application of this principle, but I can only find it unattributed in two websites. The story is basically similar in both; here is one of the two similar versions that I could locate, followed by references to the websites:

Once there was a man, who lived in a house and had a lawn. And kids would come to play on this man's lawn to have fun. The man began to be annoyed by this, and decided to do something about it. So, strangely enough he paid them a dollar to come and play on his lawn. The kids happily took the dollar and played on his lawn. The next day, the man told the kids that he did not have enough money, so he could only give them 50 cents to come play on his lawn. On the third day, he told them he could only give then a nickel to come play on his lawn. The kids were displeased with this, and told the man he could forget that, and that they would not play on his lawn for such a cheap reward. What happened? These kids played on his lawn before for absolutely nothing, but now, they quit playing, even though they were offered a nickel! Well, it just so happens that this man understood an important concept... That is, the effects of external rewards on intrinsic motivation[8]

It may be necessary to get the child or adult to perform some action that they would not ordinarily want to do, but for intrinsically interesting things such as drawing, playing or, by extension, learning new ways of thinking, then these external rewards are damaging. Playing in school should be a major positive event. But we may well be a nation of undermined reward-seekers. Children around the world would give nearly anything to be given an opportunity to go to an American school, while our own (undermined) American children grumble and seem to dislike the experience. Where did we go wrong? We went wrong devising our public versions of the Expected Award condition, undermining intrinsic interest with external constraining rewards.

The happiest and busiest people are those who volunteer to do what they want to do; the most disgruntled and unhappy are those who are doing things because they "have to." When children complain that they *have* to go to school, or have to do their homework, then we have very suggestive evidence of the damaging effects of rewards. One could look at the history of worker-manager relationships in this same causal framework. When workers go on strike for higher pay, when teachers give children A grades, when athletes compete for Gold Medals, they are in danger of pursuing an external reward with the damaging consequences for the whatever intrinsic motivation might otherwise be present in that situation.

The implications of this basic undermining effect are quite profound. If you look around and think about the world we have built for ourselves, you will see the dangers of undermining. Without going into experimental details, here is a quick review of ways that you can see how we are undermining our intrinsic motivations in our daily lives.

- Gold stars, trophies, Oscars, gold/silver/bronze medals, etc. We all want to honor outstanding achievement, but from the performer's perspective, if they do their activities with the intent of winning honors, then they are undermined. We would expect them to decrease their activities once they have achieved their (external) goal, as opposed to achieving a chance to continue to perform their (intrinsically) motivated activities.
- Pay. Working for pay as opposed to working for the opportunity to work is the classic example of external motivation. Reduce the amount of pay or eliminate it and the performance will deteriorate or stop. This is not to deny the necessity of pay for survival, but the perception of the true reason, internal or external, for doing the performance is the key to the motivation and stability of the performance.
- Surveillance. Some bosses like to keep tabs on their employees, and some teachers maintain strict surveillance of the students in their classes. Intrinsically motivated workers and students will keep working even without surveillance, but just how common is it that "when the cat is away, the mice... just keep on working?" Disrupted classrooms and "goofing off" are more likely the consequences of workers and students motivated by the gaze of the "higher authority."
- To make an impression. People dress nicely, do their hair, nails, face, or bulk up their muscles, all in order

to give others a favorable impression of who they are. If those others do not respond as expected, this form of externallybased motivation is likely to lead to unpleasant consequences. This can lead to a frantic reworking of one's image in an endless cycle of trying to find out what others want.

- Competition. Trying to "beat the opponent" rather than trying to be the best one can be no matter the consequences is a subtle but poisonous influence on performance. An external focus on "the other" means a reduced focus on one's own skills and even one's true motivations.

- Deadlines. Sometimes we have a task, either self-chosen or imposed on us by others or by a system, which puts an externally-imposed force on us. To that extent we lose control over our own self-chosen course of action, reducing our own sense of control. Completing a task at work by a deadline, getting a class assignment handed in by the required time, getting to a public function at the announced time, are all ordinary examples of how we lose our own sense of control. There is an almost universal reaction to meeting an externally-imposed deadline: Once it is met, people tend to quit, to back off, to cease working at the task. This letdown is likely to be harmful to the overall longer-term enterprise, suggesting that imposing a deadline may not be the best course of action.

Success in Drug Treatment and School Performance

Understanding the basic logic of how undermining occurs leads you to focus on the person's interpretation of how they become motivated to perform: For internal reasons or for external reasons. Taking that logic to another level, my colleague Sara Gutierres and I[9] conducted an extensive study of the motivations of male and female drug-abusing adults, in this case clients living in therapeutic communities in Arizona and California. We were interested in finding out how drug abusers thought about the possible causes of their problem. We also wanted to link up their thoughts about their drug abuse with how successful they were in their ongoing treatment and their perceived success or failure to gain from their treatment. Succeeding at drug treatment should be a major positive event.

We recruited a sample of 35 drug abusers enrolled in residential treatment facilities in cooperating drug treatment facilities in the Arizona and California. As a comparison sample, we recruited a sample of 76 similar-age and gender adults residing in the neighborhoods of our drug abuser sample. This was an attempt to match our two groups on demographic characteristics as much as possible, given the complexities of field research.

To assess our key responses of interest, we administered an extensive set of questionnaires assessing particularly their thoughts about the causes of their treatment experiences. We then kept in contact with them over time for a second assessment 2-4 months' later where we again asked them to provide causal accounts for their treatment experiences. While some were still in treatment, others had successfully graduated out, while others had quit treatment and returned to their drug abuse. These are important outcomes, not ones we could manipulate as Lepper, Green and Nisbett did, but outcomes resulting from the naturally occurring thoughts and feelings in people experiencing "real world" problems. We queried all of the participants about their success or their failure by asking them what they perceived the causes to be of their current status.

Our results were consistent with what you might expect from an intrinsic motivation/undermining interpretation. Those respondents who were successful in their rehabilitation rated that their success was due to their own efforts rather than to some external reason. For instance, they rated higher on the item: "Have experienced an awareness that I am able to quit using drug and improve my life." However, those respondents who failed in their treatment tended to choose an external reason: "Friends and/or a boyfriend/girlfriend had a significant influence on my beginning to use drugs again" (for "failure in treatment" respondents). While many forms of drug treatment programs are focused in raising the self-esteem of their clients, this model suggests that the attributions of causation of their success or failure in treatment is a particularly valuable way of looking at treatment effects. Clients can get undermined in their motivations if they believe that the causation for their treatment is residing in others rather than themselves. But they can increase their chances of successful treatment if they internalize positive goals and motivations and come to see them as under their causal control, as Lepper, Green and Nisbett might suggest.

Volunteering and Caregiving: Ways to a Longer and Better Life

Undermining motivation by external control has powerful effects, and it appears that turning play into work is apparently fairly easy to do: Switch the person's motivation from internal to external, and pay is the classic distractor to do that, and you are setting up a decrease in internal motivation. But there are situations in life where pay would be an unnatural occurrence. Mother Teresa, for instance, needed funds to maintain her health clinic in India but had no interest in money for herself; she worked simply for the intrinsic desire to help the underprivileged. Indeed, throughout the world we see people helping others with no motivation for pay. The healthcare system, for instance, has its financial side: Paying staff, maintaining expensive facilities, training future physicians, but this overlooks the millions of family members who care for their ill spouses and children, and the large number of people who volunteer of their own personal choice to donate their time and effort to hospital activities with no external reward involved.

This is all very reminiscent of the Fredrick Herzberg "motivator factors" which I discussed in Chapter 3. Even more, the entire realm of non-profit organizations, so important to our local and national social services, relies heavily on informal care through unpaid staff for their operations. Billions of dollars of potential costs never have to be reimbursed to maintain and improve the welfare of individuals, communities and nations around the world because the people who fulfill those needs are not motivated for pay; they are motivated by intrinsic desires to help others. The data I will present next show that they are in fact helping their own welfare as well.

Personal Improvement through Freely-Chosen Actions

Taking this book's perspective on things, if volunteering is a form of a desirable event under the personal control of the person then we would expect positive benefits to derive from freely-choosing to engage in volunteer activities. There is evidence that volunteering time and effort to help others in fact is beneficial both physically and emotionally. Stephanie Brown, Dylan Smith, Richard Schulz and others in their research team[10] conducted a statistical analysis of a national survey of over 3,000 community-dwelling older adults and their spouses. There were 4 repeated surveys, allowing an assessment of mortality over time. The participants responded to questions concerning how much help was provided to the spouse (and how much help the spouse reported receiving). The data were fine-grained such that the investigators could calculate the number of hours per week help was given or received. With other variables such as physical health, age, race, employment status, *etc.* controlled in the statistical analyses, the results showed that those participants who gave more help actually lived longer (experienced significantly lower mortality) over the 5-year period of the study. In spite of the strain of caregiving, if helping someone is considered in the context of the spousal care situation, helping that spouse is linked with lower mortality. The investigators link that helping behavior to compassion and they argue that helping others buffers the stresses of the illness and in fact may well strengthen the caregiver's immune response system.

Interestingly, in a related study by Brown, Randolph Nesse, Amiram Vinokur, and Dylan Smith,[11] it was found that, while giving help to others was related to lower mortality, being the one who is helped, *receiving* help as opposed to giving it freely, did not improve mortality figures. Being helped was in fact shown *not* to be helpful in terms of extending life. Being in a condition of needing help and actually receiving it may be due in part to being in a dependent situation, having to rely on the external control by others rather than oneself. I will discuss this issue of receiving help again in Chapter 7.

Caregiving itself in this context can be separated from volunteering as in joining and helping out organizations. Morris Okun, Kristin August, Karen Rook, and Jason Newsom[12] showed, again, reduced mortality even among volunteering adults 65 years and older who had problems with their daily functioning due to health limitations. Other research such as that of Elizabeth Midlarsky and Eva Kahana[13] has shown that volunteering is associated with older adults' sense of competence and higher levels of being in control of their life's events. These data are interesting because they provide a sharper analysis of personal mastery and control processes. The fact that volunteering has been shown to have such broad-band positive effects is excellent evidence for the power of personal control and freely choosing to be a help to others. And this study also shows the downside of receiving help.

Elusive Expectancies: Gambling and Playing the Lottery
In our pursuit of desirable events we naturally pursue goals that we expect will pay off in increased positive feelings.

Expectancies in our choices play out in other ways as well, often to our serious disadvantage. One of the more "fun" things to do in the minds of many people is to gamble. Betting on horse or dog races, betting on our local and national sports teams, buying lottery tickets... the list goes on and on. This lucrative business is worth billions to those who own and manage it, but the chances for the individual to make a significant gain are miniscule. The odds are stacked against the individual, and very much in favor of "the house."

So why would people engage in an act so perfectly set up for them to lose? We are back to our free choices and our expectancies again. People who gamble always hope to win, there is some degree of expectancy that they will win, and in a few games of chance such as poker their skills may in fact have something to do with their outcomes. There is always the haunting idea that "if you don't play, you can't win." So there is a built-in hope and even expectancy of feeling good. This leads to the presence of the factor of free choice. It is so easy to choose to gamble, especially if you are under the influence of the tricky mixture of desire and hope. Choosing gives it value, and as you know, choice is an exercise of our personal mastery over the game.

While some forms of gambling may require some skill and technical mastery motivations, winning a lottery is just luck. You can blow on dice and you can calculate odds of winning with cards and, fortunately, you can learn from your mistakes. But a lottery is different: You have no effect on winning or losing at a lottery. Let me repeat that: You *cannot* have an effect on winning or losing at a lottery. Naturally, that does not mean that people think that they have no effect on winning: If they were absolutely convinced that they have no effect, then their desire to gamble their money should accordingly be reduced. But clearly that is not the case: Lotteries around the world gain billions of wealth willingly contributed by people who apparently think that they have a high chance of winning. To increase their chance of winning, they will engage in various form of personal control: They will carefully pick numbers from their own life or they will rely on some other cause, something called "luck" (as in, "I hope to get lucky") in the expectation that it will get them their desired outcome.

Gambling provides us with some useful insights into the subtle power of personal control. We have to disentangle the effects of chance occurrences such as winning and losing (over which we have no control, of course) from the act of choosing to engage in the act itself. We also have to disentangle the behaviors that people will do to try to control their outcome (blow on the dice, pull the slot machine handle slowly or quickly, wearing a favorite sweater, *etc*.). People do these things, but the fundamental choice to engage in doing them is the ultimate key to understanding the power of personal choosing itself. That is a tricky but important distinction to make.

Ellen Langer of Harvard University designed a clever study in a real-world setting to parse out personal choice from the other confounding components of the gambling situation.[14] Her experimental setup was very simple. She approached employees of two companies whose employees traditionally held various drawings and cash pools for betting on sports contests. Unbeknownst to them, the participating employees were randomly assigned to two conditions. In the "High Choice" personal control condition, the respondents were asked if they wished to participate in a lottery. The cards cost $1 (that is important to remember when you see the results). If they agreed to participate, they were presented with a box of lottery cards and asked to physically choose which one they wanted and to pick it out. The type of card they chose was noted, they selected it from the box, and they were instructed to keep it themselves for the later drawing. When they chose their particular card, an identical paired card was dropped by the experimenter into the lottery box.

For the other participating employees, the "Low Choice" low personal control condition was nearly identical except for one crucial detail. In this condition, after the respondent was approached and asked if he or she wanted to enter the lottery, for those who said that they would agree to participate and paid their $1, they simply were handed a lottery card picked from the box by the experimenter; no choice of card was mentioned to them. Actually, the card was matched to the one chosen by a respondent in the high control condition, so nearly every detail of this study was identical between these two experimental conditions except the degree of control and choice that the respondents exercised.

Once this phase of the experiment was over, the tests of the effects of these two different experimental conditions were very cleverly assessed. On the morning of the lottery drawing, each respondent was approached again by the experimenter and was given the following little talk:

Someone in the other office wanted to get into the lottery, but since I'm not selling tickets any more, he asked me if I'd find out how much you'd sell your ticket for. It makes no difference to me, but how much should I tell him?

The amount of money (worth) that the person stated was the key result: How much he or she "charged" would be a direct indicant of how much he or she valued the ticket. Would valuing be based on how much personal control the person asserted in acquiring the ticket in the first place? The results for the two experimental conditions were strikingly different. The High Choice group participants charged an average of $8.67 for their tickets, whereas the no choice respondents charged $1.96 for theirs. Remember that they all paid $1 for a ticket! Although the differences in how they acquired their tickets might seem to be slight, from a personal control perspective it is obvious that those differences were in fact pretty major.

An anecdote brought home to me a bigger picture of how personal control fits into the broader scheme of a person's life, and the story involves lottery tickets. I was part of a team of lawyers and financial advisers providing a workshop for professionals on inheritance and sudden windfall gains in wealth. We gave all the attendees a small gift of a scratch lottery ticket to stimulate group discussion. However, after we passed around a box of lottery tickets, one obviously successful, undoubtedly "high powered" lawyer raised his hand and asked, "What is this?" He simply did not know what a scratch lottery ticket was. When he was told that it was a scratch lottery ticket, he then asked, "What am I supposed to do with it." "Well, scratch it to see if you won." He had to ask the person sitting next to him if he could borrow a coin to scratch it, which he did and, of course, did not win anything. His look of a combination of puzzlement and possible irritation at the disruption of the workshop schedule showed to me that, no doubt about it, he did not gain his wealth and power by relying on chance. I suspect that he kept control of his life pretty much in his own hands.

Winning In Gambling: Does It "Pay Off" in Our Happiness?

So the question becomes, when people do actually win at a lottery, what are the *consequences* of that winning? The question seems a bit silly even to ask: Of course lottery winners will be happier than non-winners (the comparison group). Why would one even ask the question? But from a personal mastery perspective, it is an important issue. Since you cannot personally cause the outcome, good or bad, even engaging in the activity is to submit oneself to an "out of control" experience. It is logically possible, therefore, to experience negative consequences from winning even though gaining the new money will be a nice thing. There is no question that not winning will be unpleasant, but even at that there are, logically, two ways in which losing will have poor consequences: (1) The disappointment of a loss and (2) the distinct knowledge that your attempt at controlling your outcomes failed. We know from the economics research of Daniel Kahnemann and Amos Tversky[15] that people dislike losses more than they value gains. Any financial loss should hurt. But I would add that the psychological significance for one's sense of loss of being in control of one's outcomes is perhaps equally if not more powerful than not gaining the money.

At any rate, lottery gambling is a particularly interesting case of the complex linkage between a desire for money, choice and a motivation to maintain and enhance one's sense of mastery in life. This issue was investigated by Philip Brickman, Dan Coates, and Ronnie Janoff-Bulman[16] working from the perspective of their Campbell-Brickman hedonic "treadmill model" of happiness which I discussed earlier in this chapter. Living in the State of Illinois at the time, they were able to track down and interview 22 people who had been winners of the Illinois State Lottery, and then to compare those winners to the reactions of 88 non-winners whom they selected from the same neighborhoods by using their city's telephone directory. Among the lottery winners, 7 had won $1 million, 56 had won $400,000, 2 had won $300,000, 4 had won $120,000 and 3 had won $50,000.

I think that most of us would automatically assume that these winners would be happier and have better lives than the matched control sample who had not found themselves with a sudden windfall of this magnitude. Interestingly, Brickman, Coates, and Janoff-Bulman made the specific prediction that the winners would *not* be happier. To get at this, in their battery of assessment questionnaires they included questions that asked the respondents, among many other measures, to rate a good sample of routine small daily events in their lives on a 6-point pleasantness scale from "not at all" to "very much." Some events to be rated were: "talking with a friend," "watching television," and "reading a magazine." The experimenters also asked the respondents to rate how happy they were with their lives in the past, now, and how happy they expected to be in the future.

As the investigators expected, the lottery winners were less satisfied with their daily events and they were not significantly different from the non-winners in the judgment of how happy they had been, were, or expected to be in the future. The winners did report on other questions that they had fewer financial worries than they used to have and that they had increased leisure time. But in their daily events and their overall happiness, they did not report feeling better off than non-winners. The investigators explained these results from the perspective of adaptation level (AL) theory; experiencing the immediate high of winning led them to become less happy; becoming more neutral about the events of their daily living. I would argue for the same effects but from a personal mastery perspective. Once you enter a lottery, your fate truly is not in your hands, so if you win, you have to know at some level that was "dumb luck" and it has nothing to do with you as a person or your sense of being in control of the events of your life. It was all external to you and therefore not very positive or satisfying. In fact, the investigators asked the winners how much control they had over the win, and 71% of their responses attributed it to chance.

Of course there is much more to the case than this, and an interesting body of research literature has built up over this finding. A number of journalists have interviewed big-time winners and found that a whole host of other problems arise when the word gets out that someone is a winner. Among other problems are the constant demands by friends and strangers for a free gift and even family members turn nasty and aggressive. Handling a large amount of money is complicated and winners often are unprepared and unskilled at knowing what to do. They tend to spend unwisely, often resulting in bankruptcy. As one workshop participant said to me, "If you win a big sum, just take your problems and add a lot of zeroes to them." So I am not claiming that loss of personal control is the only explanation for the disasters of gaining an unexpected windfall.

Let me also add several more cautions to this complicated issue. First, let me say that I fully understand that you personally may not agree with me about the downside of winning. There are always individual differences going on inside group statistics such as this study reported. Research is necessarily based on group averages, and not every person's feelings and behaviors are reflected precisely in the group's overall tendency. But that tendency is the best predictor of any given individual's reactions. There is also potentially a problem with applying the AL model of Brickman and colleagues to this issue. Adaptation to an extreme positive event may not be all that is going on in this situation. Edward Diener, Richard Lucas, and Christie Scollon[17] have reported that individuals vary in their adaptation level neutral points, that neutral points are not stable over time, and desirable and undesirable events can change in different directions over time as more experiences accumulate. Their main point is that the specific applications of the AL model are not rigidly determined by invariant processes. Nevertheless, the general idea that the emotional impact of experiences becomes less impactful over time is an important finding. If one is going to set out on a road to endlessly pursuing happiness, there are going to be a lot of potholes on that road. Also, it will have many forks in it with no guaranteed map to find your way. Your internal compass pointing toward more ways to exercise your personal mastery rather than trusting it to luck seems to be the best guide for you to follow.

Economists have shown considerable interest in lottery winning and other forms of sudden wealth acquisition because they provide data on the relationship between financial gain and well-being. They typically obtain their data from national surveys. The most recent studies again confirm no simple relationship between winning and well-being, but more complex relationships are starting to appear. For example, an analysis of a national survey of German citizens[18] did not find an immediate relationship, but repeated assessments found that, two years after winning a large lottery, participants were reporting a significant improvement in their satisfaction with their finances. Interestingly, winning a smaller amount was not related to satisfaction even after the long delay. Other investigators have found the same two-year lag, in this case in a survey of British participants who won medium-sized lotteries.[19] This time gap may be an important consideration. In another British study,[20] it was found that lottery winners started engaging in risky health behaviors such as increased smoking and social drinking, so in fact winning did change their lifestyle, but in a negative direction. The two-year lag may have helped the participants adjust to the stresses of handing their sudden financial gains. This study also showed a reduction in measures of stress such as anxiety and depression, but the original surveys in all of these studies did not contain positive outcome measures such as happiness or optimism about the future.

The issue remains somewhat murky. But there is little or no evidence that you should expect to see a sudden burst of positivity in your life if you choose to gamble on the lottery. Winning a lottery is not exactly a perfect example of total external causation, since we spend some money to buy the ticket and we spend a good deal of time dreaming about how we would live if we had that big golden gift descend on us. We tend to take (causal) credit for positive things in our lives, and so we would value the winnings as if we had actually made them occur. There are ways other than gambling that this can occur. The question is, then, what is the outcome when we suddenly gain an unexpected windfall of, in this case, money? That question was almost inadvertently answered by a personal experience reported by Hal Arkes, Cynthia Joyner, Mark Pezzo, and Jane Gradwhol-Nash.[21] They conducted a research study on the "spendability" of anticipated and unanticipated windfall gains. They described a story they had heard from a woman who had participated in a large publishing company's annual employee retreat to the Bahamas. The company distributed bonus payment to all of the employees a $50 cash gift. The gift was completely unexpected and all were pleasantly surprised.

Perhaps unfortunately, it turned out that there was a gambling casino near to the hotel headquarters where the employees were staying. The investigators led off with the story of "Nancy," one of the employees who spent her entire $50 gift there, as did most of the other employees. But the important point of this story for our purposes is how Nancy later expressed disappointment about her spending the money:

> If I hadn't been given the $50, there's no way I would have spent a dime at the casino. There are plenty of things I could have used that money for. Why did I waste it? (p. 331).

In their more controlled, rigorous studies on the effects of unanticipated gifts *vs.* anticipated gifts, the investigators engaged their participants in games with either type of situation, then they had their participants rate how they would spend their rewards. Nancy's personal story was supported by the actual outcomes of 5 experiments. People are much more casual and wasteful with money they received but did not anticipate, but if they saw the gifts as expected results of their efforts, they were significantly less wasteful.

There is a principle here: Anticipating something is a process whereby we draw a causal connection between our efforts and our outcomes. In that sense, we come to value what we willingly choose to do, and consequently we value our outcomes and the results show that we downgrade the value of that windfall. Given Nancy's apparent anger or disgust with herself, you have to wonder if there might be something rather harmful about her sudden windfall gain. Was her self-esteem worth $50? Isn't our positive regard for ourself (our self) one of our most precious possessions?

There have been a number of other approaches to the issue of the wealth/happiness relationship, and it has been consistently found that there is little connection between the two. Interested readers might want to trace out other explanations, a number of which are summarized in a review by Daniel Kahnemann, Alan Kruger, David Schkade, Norbert Schwarz, and Arthur Stone's paper in the journal *Science*.[22] In general, the bulk of the research literature would certainly discourage people from assuming an automatic connection between obtaining wealth and obtaining happiness. The key is to see the pursuit of both to be an exercise of our own personal control. Playing cards such as poker do reflect some levels of skill and experience and therefore are excellent examples of personal choice and exercising our sense of control. But picking a scratch lottery ticket, no matter how big the prize, has little benefit for your sense of competence and mastery.

The Power of Rejecting Choices

You can stop yourself from gambling, although it is not necessarily an easy thing to do. In general, most of us are in nearly complete control of a big portion of our daily living, and we exercise that control so often, so habitually and automatically, that we do not have any consciousness awareness of doing it. It is like a fish in water; the last thing the fish would note, if asked to describe its world is that it is composed out of water. We know that losing control has wide-ranging harmful effects, and we know that gaining control has helpful consequences, even if it is just the thought that we can control things, such as Glass and Singer[23] showed with their "control button available but not actually used" results.

Being in the habit of controlling our daily events has the advantage of making us function quickly and efficiently during the day. But since it is so common, we are alarmed when we have to face those occasions when our control is threatened. Perhaps these occasions magnify our worries and concerns about control, even to the point that we come to think that our lives are slipping into helplessness and depression. Indeed, having a sense of lost personal control is thought by clinical psychologists to be a key component of clinical depression. The learned helplessness research of Seligman and Maier certainly supports that interpretation. Losing control over positive events has a downside as well.

Given that, then decisions we make about alternative paths to take in our lives can become central to our mental health. But we have to think carefully about just what is involved in making decisions, both about major life events and the smaller daily events of our lives (which my colleague Alex Zautra and I call "demands" and "desires"). You might be amazed if you took time out and not just how many choices you make during the day. Some of these might be major, important and possibly stressful or uplifting, but many of them will be small and more habitual in your daily routine. So if you can become more aware of all of the choices that fill your life, you will be able to see how your personal mastery is reflected in the decisions you make. I suspect that you will be surprised to discover how much personal control you are expressing as a matter of daily routine living.

Let me put this into practice by giving a research example and then explain its underlying control principles. In 1983 Lawrence Perlmuter and Ellen Langer[24] selected a small sample of male retirees living in the Boston area and recruited them into a study assessing the effects of some relatively simple instructions about how choices affect the degree of control people feel in their lives.

They divided the residents into three experimental subsets and gave each group a slightly different task to do for the following three weeks. All were to monitor their daily activities by focusing on what they chose to do each day. One group, the "Regular Behavioral Monitoring" group, was asked to focus on just one behavior, choosing the first beverage of the day, and then, each day, to answer 3 simple questions about it: What it was, how much they consumed, and how much they enjoyed it. Group 2, the "Varied Behavioral Monitoring" group, were asked to monitor a *different* activity each day, for example, choosing a beverage, what color shirt they decided to wear that day, what TV program they watched, *etc.* and to answer the same 3 questions. Group 3's instructions differed significantly. This group, the "Rejection Behavioral Monitoring" group, was like the Varied Behavioral Monitoring group, except in this case they were to list three activities each day which they might have chosen but instead decided *not to do.* They were to pay attention to what particular activities they had considered but then actively chose not to do.

After their 3-week monitoring period, all of the respondents were brought together for a general discussion of their experiences. Importantly, they also answered a questionnaire to provide more specific information on their reactions to the experience in terms of sense of personal control. The results showed that the Rejection Behavioral Monitoring group outscored the other groups on measures of perceived control over their daily experiences. Perlmuter and Langer suggested that choosing to reject alternative courses of action led the participants to generate thoughts which they otherwise would not have considered, thereby enhancing their sense of control. Considering choices available to us is a form of decision-making which is more effective than just choosing and doing, *per se*. Note that there was no strong attempt to make the respondents change their actual patterns of living but just to pay attention and monitor their daily living pattern, raising consciousness of the alternatives that they have considered. It is empowering to think of what you might do and then consciously, deliberately choose not to do it. This finding is a key to the self-management project I will discuss in my last chapter's description of our personal mastery intervention project.

In Sum

We all want happiness in our lives, and we often make a lot of effort to increase the amount that we have. The beliefs that we have about that goal, and the actions we take to achieve it, are more complicated than might initially appear to be the case. The personal mastery perspective suggests that it is possible that we are sometimes making mistakes in that quest. The Brickman and Campbell adaptation-level model (AL) proposes that having continuously desirable experiences, *per se*, will fail because of the futility of trying to beat the hedonic treadmill. But that model, while compelling in and of itself, does not account for personal control processes: The research I have discussed throughout this book clearly indicates that we can experience significant levels of satisfaction and well-being by creating for ourselves, from our own personal mastery resources, positive events which we cause to happen.

But pursuing desirable events under the assumption that they will automatically make you happy is not necessarily a winning strategy. Events not under our control can lead to less satisfaction in life, even if they appear superficially to be desirable. Winning a lottery, gambling, taking a $50 gift from your boss when it is not personally deserved, even entering a drug treatment program because your family wants you to, all have been shown to have negative side effects. Gifts may be free, but there is a cost to them in terms of what you believe about your own personal mastery.

Our choices play a key role in how the mechanics of these quests for positive experiences play themselves out. When you choose to pursue a positive event, your choice automatically gives that decision a power over your own sense of mastery; choices are indeed tricky. But you also have the freedom to reject a choice, and rejecting choices is in and of itself an exercise of your mastery. As Perlmuter and Langer showed, even as rejecting what color of shirt to wear can increase your sense of control in your daily life. While it may appear tempting to go for that free cupcake at your office coffee bar, resisting that temptation can give you strength because it is your personal mastery that is on the line. The American essayist Ralph Waldo Emerson stated this principle nicely:

We gain the strength of the temptation we resist.[25]

In these two chapters, I have now discussed the major properties of desirable and undesirable events in the context of how our personal control over them relates to positive and negative aspects of our psychological adjustment and well-being. Fortunately, investigators have taken the principles I have discussed to the next level, to the level of therapeutic interventions, where experimental tests of various techniques to enhance personal mastery have proven successful at enhancing the well-being of participants in those interventions. In the next chapter, I will discuss specific details of how those interventions were developed and implemented. In turn, those discussions will prepare you for adopting those principles yourself as they are demonstrated in the experimental project my colleagues and I developed as presented in my final chapter.

Chapter 6

Intervention Projects Enhance Well-Being

As you will recall, in Chapter 2, I reviewed some studies which defined personal mastery as a trait, as a relatively stable, enduring personality trait of the person, along with some sample items from the various questionnaires which are traditionally used in assessing that trait. Scores on these instruments validly predict positive and negative physical and mental health outcomes. This particular domain of personality assessment has been one of the most productive areas of psychological research. One major issue about this approach to personal mastery deserves more in-depth discussion. It is an open question as to how malleable our beliefs in our personal mastery really are. Technically, in psychological research, traits of personality are treated as stable, enduring, and generalized across time and situations. As such, we would have to predict that they would not be changeable. But given how useful it is to have high levels of personal mastery, it would seem to be personally and societally useful if we could find techniques which can increase one's personal control.

One thing we know about our sense of personal mastery is that it is closely attuned to our environment of controllable and uncontrollable events. My review of the PXE congruence model showed a close connection between our personal control and our ability to manage our life's events and their outcomes. Finally, in Chapter 5, I showed that the act of choosing, our exercising of our personal choices among available alternatives, is the key linkage between our internal personal mastery beliefs and the external world.

In this chapter I can now move us up to a new level where it has been shown that we can actually enhance personal control beliefs and actions. The operating principle is that by giving people awareness of how they make choices about their events and their causal effects on their environment, then they can gain an important insight into how their personal control beliefs match, or do not match, their environment of events. A good "fit" or match can improve their well-being. As you will see with the research examples I want to present in this chapter, you yourself can enhance your personal mastery by gaining more and better control over the events you experience. This type of approach is the key to personal empowerment which is the central aim of the personal mastery line of research and therapy.

Literally dozens of psychotherapies and mental health programs have been developed over the years in psychology, psychiatry, social work, counseling, family therapy, pastoral counseling, *etc*. Many of these interventions have been tested in one way or another for their effectiveness, and the ones that have proven to have a positive effect for people then have become part of the realm of standard therapeutic practice. As you will see in this chapter, personal mastery treatments have passed this kind of test.

It will help me to discuss personal mastery interventions if I take a moment out to describe briefly the standards used to demonstrate any treatment's effectiveness. The research approach is to select at least two samples of participants, provide the therapy of interest to one of them and withhold the therapy from the other or provide some alternative experience for the duration of the study, and then see if the first group has improved on some measure more than the comparison condition(s). Of course, there are a number of necessary methodological considerations to insure validity of the technique which need not be discussed here. But the accepted therapies show improvement in those receiving the treatment compared to the non-treated controls. The personal mastery intervention literature generally follows the same methodological procedures. As you study them, you will see that these approaches invariably involve two particular components:

Perceptions and beliefs of being a causal agent in your life.

Believing that you yourself are responsible for the events you experience, even undesirable ones, pays off in many ways, physical and mental, over the longer-term. Opposed to this is believing that you have been a passive recipient of your experiences, and research shows this belief is related to poorer outcomes. Giving research participants a button to shut off a controllable aversive noise leads to better frustration tolerance even though the button is never used; this effect is based on belief alone. On the other hand, medical patients can experience better health outcomes if they do not try to control their (uncontrollable) disease but if instead they believe that they can control their symptoms. Again, this is a matter of belief, independent of any particular actions.

Engaging in deliberate behavioral activation.

Encouraging the person to actively engage with, create, and deal with the events of their environment is related to better adjustment. One of the major comprehensive reviews of the research base of the most popular and most influential therapy today, cognitive behavioral therapy, has concluded that the main component making it successful is its focus on behavioral activation.[1] Actively doing positive, self-chosen activities leads to better mental health, especially if recently you have been experiencing a significant amount of stress. Your desirable activation can buffer you from stressful experiences.

In the remainder of this chapter I will present brief descriptions of some of the main examples of personal mastery interventions. I will start with one you already know, the "origin-pawn" studies of Richard DeCharms (see my discussions in chapters 3 and 5 for more details of his approach.)

Making People Origins and Pawns

One of the first explorations in how people can be taught how to increase their personal control was conducted by Richard DeCharms.[2] His work was important to the work on event causation that I conducted with my colleague Alex Zautra which I discussed in Chapter 3. Working with the St. Louis school system, DeCharms enlisted the aid of a group of high school teachers to participate in a training program which was structured to increase their sense of mastery. He theorized that humans have a basic motivation to be *effective*. We have a motivated drive to actively change our environment rather than being merely passive recipients of environmental events. We strive, he believes, to be "causal agents," something he called "personal causation." According to his model of the mind, we seek to be origins of our experiences, not pawns to whatever occurs. He did this work in the early 1970s, and you can see that this thinking infuses nearly everything in the research I am citing in this book (much of it starting at about the same time as his research).

DeCharms put his model into practice by developing an experimental technique for actively creating origin and pawn experiences. What makes his work appealing is that he engaged his participants in playing with model toys, an involving experience for his high school student participants. To create origins and pawns, he instructed his research participants to build two models using the children's game of Tinkertoys. All students were to build both models. One model was to be built more or less from scratch while the other was to be built according to strict, step-by-step instructions. The first condition was the "origin" condition and the second was the "pawn" condition.

In the origin condition, DeCharms provided a photograph of what the final Tinkertoy model was to look like, but he told the students to build it any way that they chose; in effect, they had complete personal control over the construction process. In the pawn condition, however, he gave the participants a printed diagram of the model and a list of nearly 50 single-step instructions to follow in order to build the model. For instance: "1. Place one red rod in a center half of a regular spool." 2. "Place one blue rod in a radial hole of a regular spool." The instructions as he presented them to the participants were not orderly and logical, however, so that the students would not be able to work on their own to build the model: They had to depend on the instructions step-by-step to complete the job. In this treatment condition, he tried to eliminate as much as possible any personal causation processes in the participants, whereas they had almost complete personal causation in the first condition.

When the projects were completed, DeCharms was interested in determining what the students thought about their experience. He assessed their personal reactions to it by a series of questions in which he had them rate their feelings about building each model. He also included a subtle behavioral technique to see if the Origin or Pawn experience had any real behavioral effects.

As you might expect from our personal mastery perspective, he found that the students' attitudes toward their experience were much more favorable in the origin condition than in the pawn condition. In that treatment condition, they reported that they felt freer in building their model than they felt in the pawn condition. He also asked them which model they would prefer to continue to work on; they rated the origin model higher. Finally, in a clever idea, when the students had completed the initial construction task, they found out that a piece of the model had been left out, a nice colorful fan which could be attached to one of the gears or an incomplete and rather ugly fan. The great majority of the students chose to add the elegant fan to their origin model, and add the ugly, incomplete fan to their pawn model. They showed a distinct preference to enhancing their self-caused model, while treating the pawn model rather poorly.

This study gives us a view of behavioral activation that is very suggestive of the power of personal control. In both conditions, the participants were to engage in actions to achieve their goals, in this case building the two models. But while the participants were equally active in the behavioral sense we are using it here, the *cause* of that activation was very different, with very different consequences. When the activity was grounded in self-chosen motivations, it had much more positive consequences for the final product. When the activity was merely following (external) orders, behavior determined by the rules of the experimenter, then the participants got less personal satisfaction out of it and they denigrated their externally-caused product adding the rather shoddy new fan to their model. To be a pawn undercuts what otherwise could have been a personally-involving and creative activity.

DeCharms next extended his ideas about personal causation to a study in a "real world" setting[3], actually going into the St. Louis, Missouri school system and training teachers in origin and pawn ways of thinking and acting. In cooperation with the system, he recruited a sample of 6th and 7th grade teachers into a 3-year training project. One half of the teachers were assigned randomly to receive origin training and the other half, the comparison group, received no special training. (Given what his other data had told him, it would have been unethical to try to create a state of pawnness, so "untreated controls" provided the necessary comparison data to interpret the result of his origin training condition.)

The original training condition involved a series of special training sessions in which he explained the origin-pawn model and he gave the teachers special exercises in such activities as the model building task. He also gave them writing assignments which he scored for originness and pawness imagery and thoughts. Overall, it was a broad-based training experience covering a number of facets of personal control thinking and action.

The results were intriguing. As you might expect, the teachers' outcome responses showed that those who had the origin training increased in their sense of originness, while the comparison sample showed no significant change. But DeCharms also discovered a truly remarkable finding. Again with the cooperation of the school system, he assessed the academic performance of the *students* of those teachers. He found that those students whose teachers had the origin training experience scored higher on standard tests of academic achievement than students of teachers who had not received any special origin training. DeCharms also scored the students' written class papers for origin themes, and he found that those who had an origin-trained teacher increased in their writing skills. Even though the origin training was only for the teachers and was not presented to the students themselves, nevertheless students with origin teachers improved in their academic performance. Finally, and also impressively, the teachers who had undergone the origin training were found, later in their professional careers to have received more promotions, higher pay, and they were granted other special training opportunities from their school administrators than the regular teachers who had not received any special origin training. Of course, the school administrators did not know which teachers had been involved in the origin-pawn training, so these impressive achievements were based only on the teachers' own achievements. Their entire careers had improved as they became more origin in their beliefs and actions, and their students showed academic gains as well.

The origin-pawn model is innovative. By linking the theory that people have a strong drive to have "effectance" with training techniques in which they can actually have influence over the events in their lives resulted in an exciting new way of enhancing people's well-being. Of course, not all of our events can be origin events, and being a pawn is not necessarily an undesirable condition: It depends on the person and the situation (our PXE model again). But the groundwork for developing other techniques for influencing personal mastery was established impressively by DeCharms' pioneering work.

The "2 vs. 12" Project

The DeCharms' studies provided a clear set of results on how the causes of our actions, our origin motivations *vs.* our pawn motivations, could be integrated into an event-based approach to studying adjustment and well-being. My colleague Alex Zautra and I undertook a study directly addressing the issue of behavioral activation.[4] Although it had been known that experiencing a greater amount of positive events is related to better mental health, research had not clarified the role of the person actually *causing* those events to occur, a more rigorous test of behavioral activation. After all, desirable things can happen to us without our own efforts, such as "receiving a compliment" or "seeing a beautiful sunset." Any favorable effects, then, could either be due to just the general glow from positive events, or from the positive benefits of being in personal control of their occurrence. This called for a study of a direct intervention to have people personally cause positive events in their lives and then assess the outcome of those event causal activities.

The study was conducted in multiple phases. First, all of our college student volunteer participants responded to a set of questions assessing their prior recent history of positive and negative daily events and also how pleasant and how stressful their lives had been recently. They were then randomly assigned to one of three experimental conditions:

- From a list pre-assessed provided by the experimenters, they were to pick out two positive events that they had not recently experienced and spend the next two weeks actually doing those events;
- Pick out from the list 12 of the positive events to do in the next two weeks, *or*
- All participants including the comparison group who did not receive any special instructions were asked to return for a post-testing in one month.

In short, the participants were instructed to engage in, basically, a few positive, personally-caused events (2), many such events (12), or no instructions were received at all. Readers who want more methodological details of this study can find it in our original research article.[4]

The results showed that the "2 positive event group" and the "12 positive events" groups rated their lives as more pleasant than the comparison participants. Interestingly, they did not differ significantly from each other, showing that behavioral activation itself had positive effects compared to the no treatment participants.

But our methodology allowed a more sensitive measure of the project's outcomes. In additional analyses, we took into account the number of stressful negative events that the participants reported experiencing before they began their participation which they had reported in the "pre" questionnaire. We found that those participants who had been experiencing many stressful events prior to the experiment but who engaged in the high behavioral activation condition (the 12-event group) reported significantly less distress at the second assessment than the 2-event group. In this comparison, the 2-event and no instructions control groups did not differ from each other.

So engaging in some positive events, no matter how many, significantly improved their participants' ratings of the current pleasantness of their lives, but the total number was not significant. However, engaging in a larger number of self-caused positive events was in fact superior at eliminating the effects of *prior* stressful events; apparently just doing 2 such events was not sufficient to raise the participants' ratings of their well-being over and above the comparison group. But the high (12) positive event experience did have a significantly more favorable effect in the context of a more stressful life. In this sense, becoming behaviorally active by deliberately increasing your positive experiences *buffers* the effects of previous negative experiences. Increasing your origin activities in bad times does have positive benefits if you perform at a higher level of self-chosen positive event activation.

We regarded this study as a "proof of concept" study, in that we showed that it was possible to separate out the positive/ negative quality of a life event from the person's own personal role in creating that event. However, it was instructive that we could improve the pleasantness of their lives with either 2 or 12 experiences, but that it took the stronger "dose" of 12 event experiences to adequately reduce any separately assessed unpleasantness that they had been experiencing. It seems clear that DeCharms was on to something very effective with his origin-pawn concept, and we were able to implement it successfully in the relatively simple two-week intervention experience that we developed.

The "Personal Projects" Study

These encouraging results confirmed our model of personal event causation. It opened up the possibility of developing a more comprehensive approach for helping people obtain a more integrated lifestyle revolving around the basic principles of event causation. We expanded our model in a later study by helping people develop a greater sense of personal mastery of positive *and* negative daily events in their lives. This helped to develop a more realistic test of personal control theory. Also, we thought that separating assessment of positive states such as positive emotions, self-esteem, and strong and supportive social bonds from the separate effects from more negative feelings such as distress, anxiety, and feelings of demoralization resulting from undesirable experiences would give us a more precise view of the project's effectiveness.

To test our ideas, we recruited 98 adults from a larger, multi-month ongoing survey of the mental and physical health of Phoenix, Arizona residents. They had been selected for that study because they had reported recently experiencing one of two major stressors of adulthood: A physical disability or the recent loss of a spouse. These conditions allowed us to have a realistic assessment of negative, externally-caused major events. Once the participants had agreed to participate in our study, we randomly assigned them to one of three experimental groups. These groups were to be guided in their personal mastery enhancing conditions in which they would be run by our team of trained personal mastery staff: (1) The experimental contact group, (2) a placebo contact group, and (3) a non-contact comparison group. Before the contacts began, the participants responded to a series of standardized questionnaires assessing positive and negative aspects of their mental health and well-being. They answered them again 6 months after the conclusion of the experiment, giving us a good assessment of pre-post changes in their well-being due to our experimental treatments.

A special group of 7 highly skilled intervention staff were recruited from the Phoenix area and given special training in both personal control concepts and of course in the technical details of how the intervention itself was to be conducted. The participants themselves were each assigned individually to one of these staff members who were to conduct the intervention person-to-person in the participant's home for a total of 4 of the experimental sessions. Readers who want more details of this experiment can find them in our report on the study.[5]

The participants were randomly assigned to the personal control condition or to one of two comparison conditions. The Placebo Contact condition involved the intervention staff person meeting with the participant for the same amount of time *per* meeting and the same timing of meetings as in the experimental treatment group, keeping experimental conditions as similar as possible. However, the staff person was explicitly instructed to not mention daily events or personal causation issues. These sessions were intended to be friendly, engaging, and pleasant interactions, but skirting entirely any of the concepts involved in the main experimental condition.

The third condition, the No Contact group, never had any meetings at all with the intervention staff person: They simply answered the same questionnaires, pre and post, that the other participants answered and at the same time as the other two groups. This condition checked for the stability of the measures over time and to control for any extraneous cultural or social happenings that might have inadvertently influenced the main participants' responses. All of the participants responded to various measures of well-being after the conclusion of the intervention phases of the experiment. This provided important "before and after" assessment of the effectiveness of the intervention conditions.

As for the intervention condition itself, it was structured as a 4-biweekly session experience with each session designed to fit within a conceptual model of how daily events have their own particular causal properties and outcomes. The first session was introductory, raising the participants' consciousness about daily events and their personal reactions to them, followed by three more specifically-targeted sessions.

- *Personal Project # 1: Examining Personal Choices.* The purpose of this session was to raise the participant's consciousness about the nature of positive and negative daily events and how we have causal control over some events and how other events arise independently from our own personal control (this is the language of "desire" and "demand" events that I discussed in Chapter 3). The staff member conducting the session brought decks of specially-prepared cards printed with examples of *both* types of events, and the participant was encouraged to generate her own personal examples. The decks of provided examples and self-generated examples were left with the participant to go over and work through daily in the following two weeks.

- *Personal Project # 2: The Happiness Project.* This session focused on desirable, positive event activities and how increasing your self-initiated activities can reflect one's choices and personal control. Again, decks of stimulus cards with descriptions of positive events were reviewed by the staff person and the participant and new cards for recording the participant's own personal choices could be created working together with the staff aide. This made the set of events very personal and relevant to the participant's own life. The participant was left with instructions to review the deck daily during the coming two weeks.

- *Personal Project # 3: The Coping Project.* This session was devoted to reviewing how external events not under our personal control arise and put pressure on us for coping. Such events tend to be negative in that they create some stress until they get resolved. This session was devoted to becoming aware of the nature of such events and learning to deal with things that we cannot control. Again, decks of cards with examples of externally-caused events were provided and the participant was encouraged to provide her own examples. This deck was left with the participant as a daily exercise to review during the coming two weeks.

- *Personal Project # 4: Balancing Happiness and Coping.* This final session was designed to last for 4 weeks. Its focus was to help the participant integrate the thoughts and activities from the prior 3 sessions into a new, balanced lifestyle. The goal was to pay attention daily to dealing with both self-caused and externally-arising events and to attempt to achieve satisfaction with the outcome of experiencing self-caused positive events and satisfaction with personally coping with externally-caused events. It was explained that it would not have to be an exact 50-50 balance, but that at least some time each day should be spent on dealing with one's desires and one's demands. Again, decks of cards with both examples were left for the participant's reviewing each day.

Several results of this experiment are of interest to us here. The main comparisons were to check on the effects of the personal mastery condition against the Placebo contact condition and the No-contact condition. Then we wanted to test for longer-term effects by assessing the results over time.

First, over the course of the 10 weeks, the participants reported engaging in more desirable event response, reflecting an increase in their behavioral activation. Also, they reported less psychological distress and negative emotions over the course of the sessions. Interestingly, the separate personality measure of personal mastery beliefs of the participants did not show any increase in the measure itself; their preexisting mastery beliefs were stable over time, as you might expect from a stable personality measure such as we employed in this study.

In a second wave of analyses of the outcomes of the study (reported separately in Reich and Zautra[6]), we found that in fact those participants who had higher degrees of personal mastery before the intervention compared to those lower in mastery in fact gained the most from the experiment. Over the course of the experiment, they reported greater gains in mental health compared to the control group participants; those who had relatively lower scores on personal mastery did not show as much improvement. Apparently the participants who had already integrated personal mastery beliefs in their style of living grasped more readily how to enhance their well-being; those who did not report significant initial levels of personal mastery did not gain as much receiving the treatment in the experimental manipulations.

One other significant finding is of interest. Recall that we included follow-up measures of well-being taken after the conclusion of the experiment. We found that the effects we initially found tended to wash out over time. At the final reporting period 6 months after the end of the intervention phase, our assessments showed that participants had returned to their initial levels on nearly all of the measured variables. Other studies, one of which will be discussed shortly, have found that initial intervention effects which initially can show up as positive benefits can tend to fade over time. This suggests the importance of giving a "booster shot" of personal mastery techniques. Many other forms of health interventions with people who have initial problems as our participants did have, found that some form of repeat treatment or technique to reestablish treatment effectiveness is needed to sustain recovery. It is very much like getting a refill on your prescription medication or having multiple sessions with a therapist. A "personal mastery booster shot" project sounds like a very worthwhile endeavor indeed.

The "Enhancing Personal Responsibility" Project

You will recall that in Chapter 5 I devoted a good deal of discussion to the personal-control properties of *making choices*. In terms of developing interventions to enhance personal mastery beliefs, having people work on the choices that they make and changing their sense of believing that they are responsible for the events of their lives would be a promising way to go. Whereas Alex Zautra and I provided explicit behavioral choices by having our participants pick and choose which actual events they could undertake, a different path would be to simply enhance *awareness* of the possible alternatives that in fact are available to us. Our lives are so filled with decision making that often we are not even aware of how many choices we actually make during the course of an ordinary day. This seems particularly promising when we are dealing with the small daily occurrences that arise and we just habitually and routinely respond to them. In principle, we can bring events up to our full consciousness and make the person aware of them. They can then choose which acts to engage in and which ones to ignore. Recall from my discussion in Chapter 5 of the Perlmuter and Langer studies on choice rejection: It shows that you can gain in personal control from consciously deciding not to respond to an event. So by raising awareness of choices and choice rejections, we can greatly enhance a person's sense of being in control of their life, and from helping them to see that, we would expect to see a consequent boost in their sense of well-being.

At the least, this process of enhancing awareness, *per se*, is theoretically a valuable route to enhancing our well-being. As I said earlier in this chapter, in addition to behavioral interventions, there is also a class of interventions which are targeted at enhancing our control perceptions and beliefs, as opposed to behavioral activation. Ellen Langer and Judith Rodin developed a pioneering consciousness-raising intervention to test exactly this model.[7]

You will recall the work of Barbara Felton and Eva Kahana which I discussed in Chapter 4. In residential care facilities for older adults, they assessed the degree to which the staff of those care facilities was responsive or not to dependency needs in their residents. They found, in effect, that staff was reinforcing dependency behavior. Attempts by the residents at being independent and self-sufficient were ignored by the staff; not punished or forbidden, just ignored. From the perspective of this book, it would appear to be more effective to increase rather than decrease residents' sense of personal control. A similar argument could be made from the learned helplessness perspective of Martin Seligman and his colleagues which I discussed in Chapter 4. So while a residential staff may be entirely altruistic, caring, and attentive to the well-being of their residents, that environment itself may well have unintended if not deleterious side effects by undermining personal control and beliefs in one's ability to cause the events in one's daily living.

Langer and Rodin developed a direct attack to counter these dependency effects by raising people's sense of choice in their lives. With the cooperation of an innovative administrator of a large Connecticut nursing home, two floors of an innovative residential home for older adults were assigned to one of two conditions, the "Responsibility Induced" condition or the "Comparison" condition. In the former, one day the residents of that floor were convened and the administrator delivered a speech emphasizing how much control and personal decision-making power that they had in their daily living. Here are a few excerpts from his speech to the *Induced Responsibility* group: Listen to them for the subtle ways in which he was raising consciousness about personal mastery issues as we know them in this book:

"...I was surprised to learn that many of you don't know about the things that are available to you and, more important, that many of you don't realize the influence you have over your

own lives here. Take a minute to think of the decisions you can and should be making... You should be deciding how you want your room to be arranged... You should be deciding how you want to spend your time, for example, whether you want to be visiting your friends who live on this floor or on other floors, whether you want to visit in your room or your friends' room, in the lounge, the dining room, etc., or whether you want to be watching television, listening to the radio, writing, reading, or planning social events. In other words, it's your life and you can make of it whatever you want.... Also, I wanted to take this opportunity to give you each a present." (A box of small plants was passed around and patients were given two choices to make: First, whether or not they wanted a plant at all, and second, to choose which one they wanted. All residents did select a plant.) *"The plants are yours to keep and take care of as you'd like... One last thing. I wanted to tell you that we're showing a movie two nights next week, Thursday and Friday. You should decide which night you'd like to go, if you choose to see it at all."* (pp. 193-194)

As you can tell, the major theme in what the administrator was saying emphasized that the residents were to see themselves as responsible for their daily activities. Taking a plant and becoming responsible for its care made their responsibilities even more obvious.

Now compare the impact of that speech to that given on the same day to the residents of the other floor, the Comparison group speech:

"I was surprised to learn that many of you don't know about the things that are available to you; that many of you don't realize all you're allowed to do here. Take a minute to think of all the options that we've provided for you in order for your life to be fuller and more interesting. For example, you're

permitted to visit people on the other floors and to use the lounge on this floor for visiting as well as the dining room or your own rooms. We want your rooms to be as nice as they can be, and we've tried to make them that way for you... We feel that it's our responsibility to make this a home you can be proud of and happy in, and we want to do all we can to help you... Also, I wanted to take this opportunity to give you each a present. (A nurse walked around with a box of plants and each patient was handed one.) *The plants are yours to keep. The nurses will water and care for them for you... One last thing: I wanted to tell you that we're showing a movie next week on Thursday and Friday. We'll let you know later which day you're scheduled to see it."* (p.194)

As you can see, there was a lot of similarity between the two talks, with the specific events and activities and the flow of ideas about the same in the two speeches. But the more subtle underlying messages about awareness of personal control were quite different: The first group was having their beliefs that they were responsible for and in control of their lives enhanced by the instructions, while the second comparison group was having it emphasized how much the staff was responsible for and controlling the daily events of their lives. The causation was being shifted from the staff to the individual in the Responsibility Induced group, and kept on the staff in the more traditional Comparison group.

What were the consequences of this experience for the residents? The investigators had cleverly included measures of the health and well-being of the residents that they thought would reflect changes in their sense of self-responsibility. They had the residents fill out questionnaires concerning their happiness and their activity levels before the experiment began and again in three weeks after the speeches. Also, the nurses answered detailed questionnaires about each resident's apparent happiness, their overt activity levels (such as visiting other residents, talking with staff members, *etc.*). They even measured how many residents from each group went to the movie!

On all of these measures, the Responsibility Induced group residents outscored the Comparison Group residents. They reported greater happiness, they rated that they were more active and the nurses agreed that they were, and more of them went to the movie. The condition of the Comparison group did not change significantly during the course of the study.

To test for the durability of the positive effects of the Responsibility Induced instructions, eighteen months later, Rodin and Langer[8] returned and reassessed the residents' well-being, this time in using nurses' and physicians' ratings of activity, mood, sociability, attitudes and physical activity. They also reviewed the residents' medical records to reassess their physical health. The initial intervention's positive effects tended to be maintained over a year and a half later. The Responsibility Induced group were more active in social activities, more self-initiating, and more vigorous than either of the comparison groups. They also showed a greater increase in their general physical health. After reviewing these generally very favorable results, Rodin and Langer concluded the following:

> *The long-term beneficial effects observed in the present study probably were obtained because the original treatment was not directed toward a single behavior or stimulus condition. They instead fostered generalized feelings of increased competence in day-to-day decision making where it was potentially available.* (p. 902).

Subsequent Projects Supporting the Langer and Rodin Technique

The success of this study has provided a key foundation in the modern new wave of thinking about how care facilities can be more open and flexible in allowing their residents more selfmastery. Recognizing the importance of the Langer and Rodin study, a number of other investigators and nursing home administrators conducted similar studies. By now, its general findings about keeping older adults active are standard fare. Some of the studies applying the original findings have themselves provided new insights into the power of this way of thinking about "helping people." I will briefly review some of them here.

Lee Slivinske and Virginia Fitch[9] greatly expanded the number and types of activities that the residents of a cooperating nursing home could experience. In addition to personal responsibility instructions, they were given classes providing knowledge and techniques to develop skills for achieving personal goals. These involved providing nutrition classes, physical fitness classes, and spirituality lessons. These one-hour classes were held twice a week for 10 weeks. Assessments conducted after the training sessions showed that the residents experiencing these classes, compared to control residents who did not receive them, reported a greater sense of power in their interpersonal relationships, they felt that they had more choice in their lives and they reported higher greater personal control beliefs. Note that not all of these training experiences were necessarily control-related, but there was a spread of effectiveness to the residents' overall improved perceptions of personal control.

Catherine Mercer and Roslyn Kane[10] found similar results in residents of nursing homes in Little Rock, Arkansas. In addition to the explicit responsibility-enhancing instructions, the experimental group residents were invited to participate in a resident council for planning administrative policy issues. Their ideas for the agenda were solicited and their council meeting actually was conducted. In addition to the usual results of improvement in activity level, a specific scale assessing their sense of hopelessness showed that they declined significantly in this negative condition over the course of the trials.

In a near-exact replication of the original Langer and Rodin study, George Banziger and Sharon Roush[11] provided residential care facilities residents with the opportunity to take a bird feeder (instead of a plant). But instead of a single gift bird feeder, the residents were presented with two different types from which to choose and encouraged to pick the one they preferred. After their choices were made, the feeders were hung outside the residents' windows and they were encouraged to keep the feeders filled with bird seed. The results of this study mirrored almost exactly the findings of the Langer and Rodin study, with significant improvement in the responsibility-enhanced group's compared to the untreated control group.

This study is particularly noteworthy because of what the investigators observed over and above the quantitative measures that they obtained from the participants' self-ratings and the ratings of the nurses. They found that one of the more withdrawn and unsociable residents became fascinated with the birds outside of the facility and interacted with the other residents over their mutual experiences of bird-watching. Another resident began pressuring the staff to buy a book for the residence with lots of bird pictures in it. Yet another male resident began growing sunflowers beside the home early in the summer to harvest their seeds, adding to the facility's seed supply in the fall. All of these examples were observed by the staff as truly remarkable but unplanned outcomes of the control-enhancing interventions. The effects of the intervention itself generalized beyond what the investigators were expecting, a real plus for this type of therapeutic treatment.

The "Predictability and Control" Project

One of the key components of being in control of the events of one's life is to be able to predict when and where they will occur. But that leads to the question of separating out the behavioral aspects of being able to control the occurrence of an event *vs.*

the belief component, being able to know when and where it will occur. One could make a strong argument that so-called "predictive control" is a key element in creating the positive effects of control that we have seen in all of the various positive benefits of control (and the negative consequences of not having control).

Richard Schulz[12] enlisted students in his Duke University classes to engage in an extended series of weekly visits with residents in a local nursing home. The meetings were to continue throughout the course of the university semester. The purpose of these social interactions was to determine the short-term and longer-term effects of these meetings on the well-being of the residents. The key experimental treatment was developed to manipulate the conditions under which these meetings were arranged and carried out. The interactions with the students either were under the control of the resident him/herself, or the interactions occurred in the same time and length of meeting as in the first group but were under the control of the student, not the resident. Again, this was a manipulation of the variable of personal choice.

The differences in the instructions between these two experimental conditions were subtle but very significant from a personal control perspective. In the "Visitor Control" condition, it was the resident's responsibility to arrange the time and duration of their meeting with their paired student. At the time those meetings were scheduled, and for the same length of time, another resident in the "Predictability" condition met and interacted with a student visitor but they did not have any control over the time and the length of the meeting; they were informed of the scheduling of the visit by the home's staff, an "external" (no choice) scheduling. This sample of residents had exactly the same pleasant interactions as the Visitor Control group but the residents only had predictability of the meeting with no actual choice over it. A third condition was similar to the first two, but residents in this group did not have any information about the meeting until just at the time that it was to happen and they had no prior knowledge of how long the meeting was going to last. A fourth group, a pure comparison group, had no meetings at all and just provided responses to the questionnaires that the other residents also answered to provide comparison data on the effects of the other experimental conditions.

To make these conditions more vivid and understandable, here are some brief excerpts the student aides followed to guide them in conducting their meetings. In all groups, the students introduced themselves to their matched resident and stated that they were "interested in having some firsthand experience with elderly individuals." In the "Control Visitor" group, from that initial introduction onward, the elderly resident was given free rein in controlling the content and length of the meetings. Near the end of the initial meeting, the student was scripted to say,

I really enjoyed talking to you. My schedule is very open right now. I can come back any time you would like me to. Do you know when would be a good time for me to come back for another visit?

In the matched No Predictability group, the student informed the resident when the next meeting would occur, stating:

I'll be at the home on (X date). I'll drop by to see you at (X) O'clock.

In the third group, the residents were visited just as frequently and for the same length of time in the Control Visitor group, with the student beginning the meeting by saying,

How are you doing? ...I decided to drop by and pay you a visit today.

The residents in this condition had no control over and no predictability in their weekly meetings. Overall, the frequency and timing of the three groups was as similar as possible given the necessity of keeping things natural, open, and friendly. The fourth group of residents provided a pure "no contact" control condition.

Schulz obtained a number of measures of the effects of this experience. In overview, the Visitor Control group and the Predictability conditions showed the most positive benefits, being rated by the residential home administrator as showing better health status and they were taking fewer medications. In their own personal ratings, both groups scored higher on "zest for life," happiness, and hopefulness. This shows that knowing that you are going to be having a positive social engagement is just as beneficial as is actually controlling the occurrence of the event. In this sense, predictability *per se* is a form of control, a cognitive form of control that has positive benefits as well.

While Schulz's study was a novel and exciting new use of personal control concepts and methods, it was a finding he obtained and published two years' later that gave his series of studies virtually classic status in the social sciences. He did what any good study should do, conducting a follow-up reassessment of the physical and mental health of the participants in the original study. His study, published with Barbara Hanusa.13 is entitled, *"Long-term effects of control and predictability-enhancing interventions: Findings and ethical issues."* The title says a lot.

Remember that the initial experiment was a one-time experience, lasting the course of the semester period for the college student visitors. At the end of the semester, the students returned to their classes and to their normal student patterns of living. But the experimenters conducted three follow-up assessments of the participants at 24, 32 and 40 months, neatly providing a "moving picture" of the well-being of the residents after the conclusion of the experience with the student visitor program.

The retirement home administrator provided ratings on general health and zest for life in the residents Schulz and Hanusa had initially assessed two years earlier. The administrator had been working the facility for nearly 11 years, so she was very familiar with the status of the residents over the course of the initial intervention and during the follow-up period.

The data were clear, but perhaps shocking: The residents who had experienced the Visitor Control and the Predict conditions *declined* substantially in their health status and zest for life over time. Interestingly, the comparison groups showed no change and no deterioration as the other experimental groups did. In overview, the groups that had gained the most in well-being as a result of their experience with the student visitors *also* exhibited the greatest deterioration in the follow-up months after the visits were terminated.

In questioning these results, the investigators noted that the experiment had not just ended quickly with no preparation. They had thought ahead of time about how the visitor contacts ultimately would have to be terminated, so they built in precautions about how it would end: The residents were told ahead of time that the formal part of the project would be over at the end of the semester, and visits were continued after the data were collected and were terminated only gradually, and the residents were told to keep in touch whenever they chose to do so. Nevertheless, these precautions did not prevent declines in the well-being of the residents. This worrisome outcome led Schulz and Hanusa to publish separately their second set of findings as an ethical and methodological warning to researchers who might be planning to conduct research on real people in real-world situations. In interpreting this result, they speculated that the residents:

...expectations for a predictable and/or controllable environment were violated by the termination of the study. Subjects' expectation for controlling or predicting important events in their lives may have been raised by the interventions used and then abruptly terminated and experimenters and visitors disappeared. This analysis suggests that the declines might have been avoided had we provided substitute predictable or controllable events. (p. 1199).

Without using the term, Schulz and Hanusa seem to be calling for a "booster shot" to reinstate a sense of predictability and control in those residents who had had their initial beliefs enhanced by the visitor program. I suggested this same recommendation earlier in this chapter. Given the significant effects of the initial program treatments, it certainly seems sound advice and it follows the best ethical standards to maintain the treatment if possible once it has been shown to be effective. Their insightful discussion of this issue is a model for anyone who attempts to enhance personal mastery beliefs or in fact any sort of intervention attempting to improve the lives of people.

Subsequent Projects Supporting the Predictability and Control Project

Another set of investigators picked up on these results. Francis Haemmerlie and Robert Montgomery[14] responded directly to the issue of improving the longer-term outcomes by making the personal control instructions more compelling. They duplicated as exactly as possible the treatment technique of Schulz, but adding in a component of a "High Salience" condition compared to a "Low Salience" condition and a No Treatment comparison group. The significant procedural difference in their study was the heavy emphasis they put on giving the residents in the High Salience condition a great deal of control over the frequency and the length of the meetings with the college student visitors. Whereas the Low Salience condition just received the visits as usual with no special attention being given to them, the High Salience residents were given explicit visitation sheets (calendars) scheduling exactly when they had set up each visitation session at their own choice, they recorded each visit by personally signing their name to the scheduling sheet, and reminders of meetings were built into the sessions.

This added emphasis on personal involvement and control paid off. Compared to the Low Salience and No Treatment control groups, the High Salience residents did not show any decrements in zest or their health status. Reassessments of their well-being at a 1-month reassessment showed no decline in their status. Even after a 1-year follow-up reassessment, they continued to show improved status on these outcomes. So Schulz and Hanusa appear to have been correct: Greater attention to firmly establishing the sense of control was shown to be effective in countering the potentially harmful effects of ending the experiment and having the visits run out at the end of the 10-week contact sessions.

In Sum

These experimental studies typically involved older adults, many of whom were experiencing the stressors of advancing age. The studies are encouraging in that they show that personal control enhancing experiences can have wide-ranging positive effects even in groups at risk for decline in their well-being. The techniques employed by these investigators differ in some respects, but the common theme is that the person can be made more aware of how their freely-made choices can lead them to handle better their own desired events while also working through their responses to events arising from outside of their own control. Without always clearly showing a direct change in their personality or their personal mastery trait structure, nevertheless control-enhancing actions were shown in these studies to lead to improvements in mental health and well-being. These studies also showed that these effects can generalize to other aspects of the person's life, above and beyond the actual experimental manipulations presented by the experimenters. Rather than giving these participants their daily fish, they learned to do their own fishing, to modify slightly the cultural truism about giving people skills for living.

The next chapter will summarize the wide range of personal mastery concepts, methods, and results I have discussed in all of these previous 6 chapters. This summary will provide a foundation for the experimental intervention study my colleagues Alex Zautra, and Mary Davis and I conducted in which we wove together into one comprehensive study the various strands of personal mastery that I have presented in this book.

Chapter 7

Opportunities and Threats to Your Mastery

Jeff Lewis's story is inspirational and his optimism and forward-lean motivation is a beacon for us all. Jeff's story is a beautiful example of empowerment in the face of what might otherwise have been overwhelming hurdles. But my purpose in presenting his story in such detail is not solely to be inspirational, but to be educational as well. There are many valuable insights into how the human mind works revealed by how he responded to his "accident." (I presume that term now means much more to you than it did before you read this book.) More, though, his story provides a living demonstration of the complexities of how people operate in their "environment of events." No one is an island, insulated from the realities of their daily events, desirable and undesirable. The research findings that I have discussed so far give compelling evidence that the characteristics of that environment *and* the characteristics of the person interact to form a new whole, a compound, a dynamic unit of action. In this compound we can find useful principles of how one's belief in mastery over the events in that environment can lead to greater levels of physical and mental health, and satisfaction in life. But there are many pitfalls in that compound as well, and I have tried to make you aware of those as well.

In the latter part of this book, I will be giving you specific, proven suggestions about how you can enhance your own sense of personal control. It will help you get into that frame of mind if I first summarize briefly some of the main results and conclusions that arise from the discussion of the research and practice literature on personal control. I began this book with Reinhold Neibuhr's Serenity Prayer, asking God to give wisdom about what we are calling in this book desirable and undesirable events. We now know that his "things" have to be defined in terms of their properties of magnitude, valence, controllability and recurrence. Given these properties, we then have the components to create our own personal template that we can apply to our own personal experiences to achieve two of life's major goals: To create desirable experiences for ourselves and others, and to try to prevent undesirable experiences from happening to ourselves and others. And if you are not always successful at achieving these goals, you always have a wide range of adaptive choices available to you; you can decide to adjust yourself to it, make an accommodation as needed, or accept that your world is sometimes unchangeable.

Now in this chapter I want to give you a short review of what we have discovered so far. My intent here is to extract from the myriad of findings from the psychological research studies I have discussed, a basic set of principles underlying how it is that personal mastery and event causation operate and have their effects on your well-being.

Mastery as a Personality Disposition vs. as Event Control (or Both)

Personal control or mastery originally was investigated as a stable disposition, a personality trait that endures and interweaves many of the person's life experiences. It is a generalized belief that the person holds about their own mastery over the events in their life. Although it is conceived of as a system of beliefs, it is not necessarily a conscious idea that you carry around at the top of your daily awareness. Maybe you will be more aware having read this book. The examples of assessment items I presented in Chapter 2 can give you an estimate of your own state of being an "internal" or an "external." I also presented research results showing the ways in which trait personal mastery is significantly related to many positive and negative aspect of your well-being.

A second but equally productive way of thinking about mastery or control is to think of it as fluctuating, as a situationbased set of beliefs and actions concerning how we handle specific events in our daily living. This way of thinking links personal control motivations closely to the environment of events in which you live your daily life. Again, personal control in the more specific sense of controlling the events of one's life has been shown in many studies to relate to physical and mental health outcomes. This approach is perhaps closer to our own conscious perception of ourselves, since it ties directly to what we see and do as we shape and respond to our daily experiences.

Demands and Desires, Hassles and Uplifts: Being an Origin or Being a Pawn

Shifting the focus to event causation in a personal control framework gives us a more precise and effective understanding of how the person interacts with their environment. We want to use the language of event causation when we try to be systematic in how we think about ourselves as we face our daily and more long-term experiences. When we are dealing with the causes of events, we can think of ourselves as "Origins" in the colorful language of Richard DeCharms when we are successful at bringing event experiences within the realm of our own personal control. My colleague Alex Zautra and I developed a related model of event causation, and we called these events "desires." Our data show that people who report experiencing more desires in their life also report better mental health. But not all events which we experience are the result of our own exercise of control: They arise from outside of us, and thus make us *Pawns*, and these "demand" events (in our language) are related to feelings of distress and lower well-being. For example, when we are having a day filled with origin events such as a vacation, then our feeling of well-being is likely to be high. But when we return to work and find the number of pawn/demand events increasing, we are likely to lose some of that positive glow. Life is a complex compounding of our demands and desires, and our beliefs and action in dealing with them.

But there are downsides to these quick conclusions. The psychological importance of the causation process is shown by the results of our studies.[1,2] As you might expect, we showed that adults experiencing higher amounts of desirable origin events also reported having a higher quality of life. But a key finding showed that experiencing a greater number of *positive pawn* events was actually correlated with poorer mental health! This also was true of negative pawn events, so it is "pawnness" *per se* and not only the positive or negative valence of our daily events that leads us to have poorer feelings overall. These studies suggest strongly that the goal of seeking positive experiences has to be tempered by how one obtains those experiences.

Types of Control: Primary Control vs. Accommodation

Directly taking action to make a desirable event occur or to do something to prevent an undesirable event from occurring are two obvious ways in which our personal mastery gets put into action. This is how we construct for ourselves the most adaptive actions that will allow us to function optimally in our lives. When we can bring the world into line with the goals, we are experiencing our *primary control*. This is a key component of the concept of empowerment which I introduced in Chapter 1.

But the world is not always so malleable. As the Serenity Prayer suggests, often we cannot get what we want and our attempts at stopping events from happening are not always successful. Such conditions can lead to learned helplessness (as I discussed in Chapter 4), appearing in such symptoms as passivity, withdrawal, emotional disruption or, in serious cases, significant depression. Since much of life's events in fact are not directly controllable by us, then it might seem that we are all inevitably doomed to end up in such states. But of course that is not the way our mind works. At our core, we are motivated to succeed in life and to conquer the inevitable hurdles that we face. When we find that we cannot bring the world into line with our desires, our mind shifts to bring our self into line with the world in the classic language of Rothbaum, Weisz, and Snyder (in Chapter 2). In fact, we have many alternative mental devices to rely on when facing an unchangeable event. By this mental route to personal mastery, we can readily accommodate ourselves if we have to, we can find ways to shift to alternative goals, and we can give up control attempts entirely and settle on a satisfying acceptance of situation.

Accommodating yourself to an uncontrollable situation can lead on to finding new paths for personal mastery, new capacities for resilience and a more realistic understanding of the world in which you are living. Jeff Lewis is an outstanding example of successfully accommodating yourself and finding a new way of achieving your goals. The act of choosing to accept the unchangeable is actually an assertion of our own personal choice and controlling actions.

In his classic play, *A Thousand Clowns*,[4] the playwright Herb Gardner has neatly characterized this possibility. In the play and in its later movie adaptation, one of the adult brothers, Murray Burns, has dropped out of the high-power New York rat race for a careless but colorful and exciting life of being as free as possible (complete self-mastery, as we would characterize it). His brother Arnold Burns (played by the always magnetic actor Martin Balsam) is encouraging him to rejoin the race, knowing that he, Arnold, looks stultified and conformist in the eyes of his devil-may-care brother. Arnold explains his approach to his own life in this riveting dialogue:

...Unfortunately for you, Murray, you want to be a hero. Maybe if a fella falls into a lake, you can jump in and save

him; there's still that kind of stuff. But who gets opportunities like that in midtown Manhattan, with all that traffic …I am willing to deal with the available world and I do not choose to shake it up but to live with it. There's the people who spill things, and the people who get spilled on; I do not choose to notice the stains, Murray. I have a wife and I have children, and business, like they say, is business. I am not an exceptional man, so it is possible for me to stay with things the way they are. I'm lucky. I'm gifted. I have a talent for surrender. I'm at peace. But you are cursed; and I like you so it makes me sad, you don't have the gift; and I see the torture of it. All I can do is worry for you. But I will not worry for myself; you cannot convince me that I am one of the Bad Guys. I get up, I go, I lie a little, I peddle a little, I watch the rules, I talk the talk. We fellas have those offices high up there so we can catch the wind and go with it, however it blows. But, and I will not apologize for it, I take pride; I am the best possible Arnold Burns…

In choosing the path of acceptance rather than futile resistance, we are able to retain our concept of our self as active, competent, and able to choose how we want to live our life. It is a second key component of empowerment as I think of it in a personal mastery framework. The personal mastery template integrating the many aspects of empowerment is displayed graphically in the next chapter, Chapter 8.

Mastery Actions *vs.* Mastery Beliefs

The distinction between personal control and mastery *beliefs* and the process of actually *making* desirable events occur or preventing undesirable ones from occurring by our actions is the core foundation of the personal mastery concept. Remember, though, that actual controlling actions are not necessarily critical to achieving desired outcomes. The Glass and Singer study[4] tested the frustration tolerance and task-solving success of research participants who were provided with a button which could cut off the presence of a noxious buzzer stimulus as they attempted to solve complex cognitive problems. Those who were given the button showed greater tolerance for the noise and better problem solving ability than participants who did not have the controlling button. That would be predicted from a personal control model of adjustment. But none of the button-condition participants actually used the button; merely *knowing* that they had access to the escape button was sufficient to give them resilience and maintenance of their adjustment capacity. A person can have self-confidence, persistence, and resilience in the face of difficult tasks if one has belief in one's personal control, even without actually exercising it.

You Can Choose to Not Exercise Your Personal Control

Personal mastery ultimately involves the act of *choice*. While it may be "natural" to choose to create a positive event for yourself, or choose not to do something to avoid a negative one, note that in both cases you ultimately have the choice to do it or not do it. Carrying out this logic, and I know it may sound peculiar, you have the power to deny yourself positive experiences! You do not have to do something, positive or negative, and not to do it is an affect and exercise of your personal choice. Many religions recommend some type of self-denial, with many variations on that theme. I suggest it here, without theological overtones, because it follows logically from our personal mastery perspective.

On the other hand, not attempting to prevent an undesirable event from occurring may well cause you even more negative events in the longer term, but nevertheless the choice is still yours. This is the core of the well-known and perhaps well-lamented condition of *procrastination*. Some people adopt it as a lifestyle choice, chronically lettings things drift along, although for other people it could be episodic and variable and particularly situation-specific. In our language of demands and desires, when demands arise, again you do not have to respond to them. Logically speaking, you can gain mastery by again choosing not to respond. But the problem with this rather peculiar sense of mastery is that the event will not "just go away" even if you wish it would. You cannot achieve very much on the basis of wishing alone. Your choice to not respond runs the risk of being self-defeating; you have chosen to let a negative event continue to exert its pressure in your life. Conversely, by responding to it, you gain in your personal mastery twice over: Once, by removing the stressful event's harmful effects from your life, and by finding one more way to assert your mastery.

Recall that Lawrence Perlmuter and Ellen Langer[5] showed that adult participants in their study reported greater control and mastery in their lives when it was suggested that they pay attention to their *choice rejections*. To face a situation in which there are several paths to take, by paying attention to what you decide *not* to do was shown to be more beneficial than just making a simple choice. In fact, Perlmuter and Langer found that participants in their study reported greater control and mastery in their lives when it was suggested that they pay special attention to the things they decided not to do. To face a situation in which there are several paths to take, by paying attention to what you decide not to do can be more beneficial than just making a simple choice.

The Upside and Downside of Desirable Events

It is a widespread belief that experiencing a lot of desirable events is a worthy goal of life. Research supports that general idea: Those people who report experiencing a greater number of desirable events in their lives also report higher levels of mental and physical well-being. The personal mastery perspective supports that common-sense approach; it proposes that experiencing those positive events is in large part due to our own personal mastery and efforts and, therefore they reflect a high level of our own personal competence and skill at optimizing our personal capacities. But not all positive events are a result of our own efforts. Sometimes desirable things just happen to us: We are given a birthday surprise party or a nice present, someone unexpectedly says something nice about us, or sometimes we (unfortunately a very small number of us) find that we have a winning lottery ticket. Although the sudden jolt of positive feelings we get from such experiences is wonderful, I suggest caution because there are problems inherently hidden in these seemingly desirable experiences.

There are two classes of such problems. One problem was raised by Philip Brickman and Donald Campbell in their concept of "the hedonic treadmill.[6]" There is an inherent tendency for our experiences to be melded and averaged into one reference point. Newer experiences then will tend to lose their emotional valence as they become merged with all of our other experiences. That is, our experiences are averaged into a middle value of neutral emotional value, the adaptation-level point (AL). To extract any positive feelings about any new experience, that experiences would have to be more positive than the AL, so it will have to be increasingly positive just to be felt as above neutral averaged base of our previous experience. To be experienced as positive, the new experiences have to be more intense or extreme in being more positive just to be felt as positive, leading inevitably to an endless hedonic treadmill and a failure to actually feel positive about those experiences. But our own research[7] shows that this effect can be overcome by increasing the number of desirable events which you yourself cause to happen. Exercising your personal mastery can overcome the averaging effects.

The second problem with externally-arising desirable events is just that: They are externally caused and therefore they do not reflect our own personal mastery. I described our research on them above, labeling them as them above a "Positive Pawn" experiences. Given their external causation, in fact, they are actually a threat to that our sense of mastery. The Brickman, Coates, and Janoff-Bulman study of lottery winners[8] in fact shows that people who win lotteries do not rate their well-being as significantly higher than non-winners. Although some studies show some positive effects of winning, overall the evidence is not compelling that winners are just automatically going to be happier than non-winners. And to think that you can make desirable events happen when sometimes you cannot is illusory. Recall my earlier discussion of the book by Sheena Iyengar, *The Art of Choice9* where she makes the point that "choosing well is the key to controlling our environment." Of course I agree with that statement, but I would add that choosing to engage in events which are under your own personal control is a key to maintaining our own well-being. By this point in this book, though, you should be wary of placing your happiness if not your very self-concept in the hands of something as out-of-(your)-control as luck or chance. What chance do you really have, anyway?

The tricky part is that circumstances can shift causation onto you such that desirable events can have very different effects depending on how they occur. A course of action much more likely to pay off is to do something where you can exercise your skills and pursue your own personal interests without external persuasion, force, or coercion. When Lepper, Green, and Nisbett10 offered their nursery school children an opportunity to play with Magic Markers, the word "play" took on an important meaning. Those who had no idea that they would be rewarded for their play engaged in it for purely intrinsic reasons, as an actualization of their own personal mastery. But those who were told that they could play if they wanted the reward being offered to them were undermined in their motivation from the start. In a later opportunity to play again, the undermined children showed less activity in playing and less creativity in their drawing. The pivot point in this study is the timing and the location of the cause of the play activity. Choosing to play simply for the fun of playing is an example of personal causation's enhancing effect on subsequent skillful performance. Internal, personal causation is the key to optimizing who we truly are, or can be empowered to become.

The Upside and Downside of Undesirable Events

In the normal course of our living, we strive to avoid undesirable events. Again, a lot of research shows that those people who report experiencing a greater number of undesirable events in their lives also report lower levels of mental and physical well-being. The personal mastery perspective supports that approach because it proposes that, generally, such events arise from causes outside of us, and therefore they signal a loss of personal control in our lives. While occasionally we may personally be the cause of such an event which we would think of as making a mistake, that is certainly not common and ordinary caution and attention and preventive effort are generally sufficient to achieve accommodation and adjustment to prevent their occurrence.

The study reported by Mirowski and Ross[11] which I discussed in Chapter 4 adds an important angle on our perceptions of undesirable events. They were able to compare people's perceptions of their personal causation of both desirable and undesirable events, comparing the effects of asserting causation *vs.* avoiding responsibility (causation) for both classes of events. The majority of participants in fact attributed high degrees of personal causation to both types of events, and that broad assertion of causation was related to lower rates of depressive feelings. Stated another way, to avoid attributing self-causation to undesirable events was related to higher reports of depression. Personal causation again was shown to be a significant correlate of better mental health. Of course, these results occurred within the confines of a controlled experiment where the instructions to the participants carefully assessed personal causation. There are limits to which this type of attribution of causation can be extended, but within the range of experiences which can be assessed experimentally, it seems clear that personal control is a powerful positive influence on our mental health.

Although we certainly do not want to cause undesirable events ourselves, that is not the full story. People who experience even major undesirable events such as serious physical accidents or more deliberately caused events such as rape have better outcomes if they can assert some form of personal responsibility for the occurrence of the event. "Blaming oneself" is not always to be discouraged or avoided: To the extent that one can find personal causation (which everyday language calls "taking responsibility") for undesirable event occurrences, then to that extent personal mastery has been affirmed. And there is no doubt that a major negative life event such as that experienced by Jeff Lewis and can be a life-changing, in fact a life-affirming, experience.

Here is what we know: In the Bulman and Wortman study of paraplegics and quadriplegics[12] and the Frazier study of rape victims[13] evidence shows that believing that we had some control over the negative event is related to better long-term adjustment. Taking "blame" in the sense of perceiving yourself as responsible for the event is a more controllable and therefore a healthier way of adapting to the experience, as bad as it is. But Frazier's research showed an important twist on the issue of blaming yourself for an undesirable experience. Good adjustment depends on what particular aspect of self-blame you choose as an explanation. If you see responsibility for your experience (rape, in this case) as due to your own causation, but as due to parts of yourself that you can change (how attentive you were, how much you were aware of the cues in the situation), then you are likely to be free to grow from the experience. This type of assertion of your personal control can help to end up leaving you better off. But if you see responsibility for the experience as resulting from stable, unchangeable aspects of yourself ("that's the kind of person I am") then attributing the experience to something you cannot do something about is going to be related to a poorer outcome and less positive adjustment.

For chronic stressors such as poor health, Affleck, Tennen, Pfeiffer, and Fifield[14] showed that to believe that you have control over the disease is related to poorer adjustment; physiologically-or medically-speaking, you do not have effective control. But believing that *you* have control over your reactions to the symptoms is a healthier course of action. Believing that *your physician* has control over the course of the disease is also a positive route to better adjustment.

There is another facet to this process, particularly in reference to uncontrollable undesirable events. When you cannot control such an event, you still have your capacity for accommodating yourself to it. We have many adaptation and accommodation routes available to us. We can change ourselves as well as changing our world, depending on the properties of the events in that situation. You can readily switch to secondary control (in Rothbaum, Weisz, and Snyder's approach to control) by accepting the condition, working to understand it, and developing new pathways for maintaining or even improving your abilities can be achieved by successful accommodation. You need not fall into a state of withdrawal, despair, or even learned helplessness. You may not be able to control the undesirable event stressor, but you can control your reaction to it. And as William James has said, paraphrasing, you can stress yourself in your own self-chosen ways, and thereby strengthen your sense of mastery and become better prepared when truly major stressors which are out of your control come your way.

The Role of Your Social Environment

A realistic view of personal mastery must certainly include the social world in which we live. Other people are a prime source of the events of our lives, embedding us in a network of constantly evolving desirable and undesirable events. The personal mastery perspective views our social relations from a specific, two-aspect angle: (1) Do other people enhance your own personal mastery beliefs and action, or do their actions undermine your own personal sense of control? (2) Similarly, when you yourself respond to other people, do you enhance their sense of control in their own lives, or do you undermine their personal control by encouraging them to be dependent on you or on other people? Let us take these two major lines of reasoning in order:

Seeking Help from Other People. First, other people's actions potentially can undermine your beliefs in your own personal mastery. It often happens that you could "use some help" in achieving a particular goal that you might be pursuing. Perhaps you are ill or sometimes you may not have the knowledge or skill that you need to solve a problem or to achieve a desirable goal. So it happens that sometimes we feel that we have to ask for help. In other circumstances, a sensitive and supportive social environment will be aware of our need and provide useful help. But this is a high-risk situation, at least from a personal mastery perspective. To the extent that the help is focused on the immediate problem to reduce the stress, or to help you obtain a desirable goal, then from a personal mastery perspective that would be considered helpful. The occasion of need can be used to (re)build your capacities and to enhance your resilience in the face of a temporary shortcoming; this can aid your return to better control over the events of your life. But if that help is aimed at overriding your personal belief that you are in control of the events of your life, such that you are encouraged to become dependent and reliant on the help-giver and not on yourself, then that "help" may well be harmful to your longer-term well-being. This is not to deny the value of short-term help for solving the immediate problem, but longer term reliance on others can lead to a decreased sense of personal mastery. The real danger is that being helped may have a spreading effect on many other aspects of your life.

In the same vein, Sara Gutierres and I[15] showed that drug abusers were more successful in treatment when they enlisted in it for reasons that they themselves felt were important. But when they enlisted because they felt that their family and friends wanted them to get treatment, then they were more likely to drop out of treatment and to show fewer signs of successful rehabilitation.

"Helping" Others. The second part of this analysis of social processes is equally complex. It is a natural tendency on your part to come to someone's aid if they need help when they ask for it or if you perceive that they need it. Indeed, this is the prototype case for children who are almost totally dependent on their social environment as they grow and develop their own control over the events of their lives. Entire professions such as the medical profession, social work, counselors, government agencies, and charities, nursing homes and volunteer non-profit agencies all swing into action. And of course we as individuals generally tend to want to help when the occasion arises. Helping others is virtually wired into us as individuals and as society. But the personal control perspective is focused on the common principles underlying control when receiving or giving help.

Although at first it may appear to be a quite different situation, the research on volunteering by Stephanie Brown and colleagues[16,17] and the work of Morris Okun and colleagues[18] find the same effects when people volunteer to help others. Playing with art drawing materials and providing caregiving help to others are psychologically equivalent from a personal mastery perspective. They reflect self-chosen acts that are done willingly and without consideration of so-called "rewards" as undermining motivations. The research shows that volunteering to help others results in better health and adjustment than receiving help.

To help someone is to run the risk of undermining their personal control beliefs, and might, therefore, have undesirable consequences. Trying to help someone by doing something *for* them may be equivalent, control-wise, to doing something *to* them. Good intentions can go awry. We may think of caregivers as giving care, but that is an iffy proposition unless we account for the care recipient's ongoing state of coping and resilience, their more stable personality disposition of being an internal or an external. After all, there are always individual differences. In this case, the fit is between the control beliefs of the person and the types of controlling help that the person is receiving from his or her social environment. In a (Western) culture which professes values of independence and self-reliance, from a control perspective we simply cannot assume that one size fits all. Some people are measurably better when they are encouraged to be reliant on others, while others can have poor reactions to being encouraged to be self-reliant. If you are in the caregiving role for another person, you now have a more complex but more sophisticated way of thinking about your social relationships. It makes for a tricky set of distinctions about helping, but the logic of the personal mastery approach is clear in its implications for how "help" may or may not actually be "helpful."

Interventions and Therapies Enhancing Personal Mastery
Although the original development of the personal mastery approach regarded it as a stable, enduring personality trait, when that framework evolved into the event control approach, it became more compatible with a model suggesting that personal

control over events could in fact be changeable. The early work of Richard DeCharms showed that, with specific types of training, people could become more "origins" in their lives rather than "pawns." A number of therapeutic interventions for enhancing one's capacity for personal mastery have been developed since then, consistently showing that such training is related to later improvements in adjustment and well-being.

These interventions generally follow two types of approaches: Giving people specific *actions* in which they can actually cause events to change (such as giving nursing home residents bird feeders) while others employ instructional sets to change *beliefs*. Both have been shown to have positive benefits on activity levels and measures of adjustment and well-being.

The Next Step

This book is based on the results of one such intervention conducted by the author and his colleagues. In the final chapter, Chapter 9, I will describe that research project in more detail, displaying graphically the results we obtained. The results are compelling and might convince you to adopt them and incorporate them into your own personal ways of gaining event control in your life. In doing this, I am following a tradition in psychological science by "giving psychology away" to the public, to cite for you one of the well-known quotations from George Miller, at the time the President of the American Psychological Association.[19] It is, or course, your choice, and I presume by this point in this book you understand how profound a statement about your personal empowerment that thought truly is.

In the next chapter, I want to give you a "take home" message covering what I am calling "opportunities" for enhancing your personal mastery and "threats" which can hinder you in taking advantage of those opportunities. It will prepare you to grasp the operating principles of personal mastery if you know ahead of time where you can find ways to exercise your mastery while recognizing ways that you might not succeed at direct control attempts. A lot of your daily events and experiences fit these two categories. To help you get the bigger picture, I will give you an organizational structure so that you can get a more systematic understanding of how all of these parts fit together.

Chapter 8

Now You Have Two Mastery Templates

Up to this point I have reviewed evidence showing the power of personal mastery as a key contributor to your health and well-being. This has involved showing in many ways how your mastery beliefs drive your thoughts and actions in the ways we define in this book: (1) striving to achieve desirable goals, and (2) striving to prevent undesirable events from occurring. But I have covered a lot of ground so far; the numerous ideas, facts and conclusions would be difficult for anyone to keep in mind as they go through their daily living. With all of this information, it might be helpful to have highlighted in one place the key elements of my take-home message about what to do to sustain your sense of mastery and personal control in your life.

You will recall that in my very opening words in my Preface, I suggested that you could develop your own personal mastery template as a framework for interpreting your experiences. In that spirit, I have devoted this chapter to two special aims. First, I want to give you a "personal radar" to "detect" control-related events in your environment and then suggest some actions you can take related to them. Some events are threats to your mastery, while others present opportunities for you to achieve your goals which you yourself set, rather than the demands that the world puts on you. The terms "threats" and "opportunities" take on a special meaning in our personal mastery framework. Then, second, I have some suggestions about the kinds of actual action you can take to enhance your well-being by applying personal mastery thinking.

By "threats" I mean the broad category of events that may in some way harm or reduce the extent to which you feel that you can control the events in your life. This means that you need to develop a systematic approach, a "template," to see how to best approach uncontrollable life experiences I call this **"Template #1, Categories of Events That Are Not Under Your Personal Control."**

By "opportunities" I mean those occasions in which you can go out of your way to find new ways to assert your personal mastery and thus create your most successful life experiences. These new ways include new controllable desirable experiences and new ways to avoid or cope with undesirable events that you yourself might cause to occur; these are most commonly called "mistakes" and we all have our own share of them. To deal with this class of personally controllable experiences, I have developed **"Template #2, Categories of Events Which Are Under Your Personal Control."**

For you to be able to integrate these concepts and the Templates into your own unique ways of thinking about your life, you need to be able to detect those threats and opportunities which are ever-present in everyone's lives. The Templates will help you do that. I will provide a number of examples of both threats and opportunities in this chapter, and I have developed a table and a graphic display of the main categories of these kinds of experiences.

I said that I had two main aims in this chapter. One was to give you a fundamental set of ideas about event control and the Templates give you a summary structure of how they can work for you. In the second half of this chapter, I carry through the logic of these Templates and I suggest ways in which you can actually apply them to some of the key ways in which you can enhance your physical and mental health: These involve proactive ways to increase your positive, desirable experiences and ways of accommodating yourself to undesirable experiences.

Given those aims, I want to remind you of the impressive insight that the founder of modern psychology, William James said many years ago which I quoted in Chapter 3. He suggested that you never miss an opportunity to stress yourself, to make your life tougher, for if you do, you will be able to stand strong when others who are trying to make life cushy and soft for themselves will fade.[1] If you make the conscious choice to engage in these assertions of control, you need to be aware of your opportunities and threats in life, and I have encapsulated them here in these two Templates.

Finding Common Ground with Other People by Applying the Personal Mastery Templates

Before presenting the details of the Templates, there is one more very useful way of thinking about them that you may find helpful; this is a rather subtle but useful side-benefit to this way of thinking about our lives. To me, life becomes more challenging and interesting if you take a personal mastery template to understanding your daily experiences. That way, you can see how your experiences, your demands and your desires, fit into a Person X Environment context. But for most of us, that context involves our continuing, daily interactions with other people; we inevitably live in a *social* context.

I suggest that we all move up a notch and look at our lives from an "external perspective." Looking at us objectively, literally as objects, you can see that all people face their lives from basically the same perspective: We all live in a world of events and occurrences which challenge or support our sense of personal mastery. Thinking objectively, we are all in the same situation, each of us facing an environment which will support or hinder our exercise of our personal mastery. Each of us applies the same Templates; you can engage yours just as they can engage theirs. With this framework, by seeing the external world to which other people are responding, you can better see where they are coming from as they try to assert their mastery in their own lives. They experience events over which they have no personal control, just as you do; and they assert their personal control to improve their lives just as you do. By applying principles of personal mastery, you can, in effect, "walk in their shoes" and see the world from their perspective. You can now see how adopting our Templates into your lifestyle gives you a dual approach: Understanding everyone's lives from the same perspective. With this perspective you can develop a rather sophisticated and, I posit, a more sensitive understanding of how and why other people act as they do. This promises to have great benefits for how we get along with others, or perhaps fail to.

An Overview of the Templates

To help you in that awareness, my two Templates will help organize the major classes of controllable and uncontrollable events which we experience in our daily living. Right now, let me briefly describe them here to give you an overview of the specific purpose I have in developing each of them. My categories in these Templates are at a general level, so naturally you will want to provide your own examples as you read them to see how many aspect of your life they detect. I will display the major category titles and then put in a few examples of each. The examples will be obvious, but seeing such seemingly-trivial events in their appropriate category should be useful in helping you see just how much of our daily living can be illuminated by a personal control perspective. This is an exercise in preventive medicine. Once you see how the Templates are developed and understand the underlying principles, you can become empowered to exercise more effective thinking and action in your daily life. The event groupings I am listing in this chapter may provide a chance to you to slow down and shift your attention more effectively to the causes of your life events, those internally caused by you and those caused externally to you, those coming from your environment.

Template #1: Categories of Events That Are Not Under Your Personal Control

You will recall this book's opening statement of the Serenity Prayer. It moves at a general level; the word "things" is suggestive but wide open for any interpretation. The personal mastery perspective employing an event perspective makes its general approach very much more helpful. To do that, we need to try to define our world of daily events and, therefore, we need to refer to our earlier discussion of event properties (presented in Chapter 3). Template #1 focuses on what we know about events that we cannot make happen, uncontrollable events. As we saw in the story of Jeff Lewis, some uncontrollable events are of major magnitude, others are smaller and more routine. But do not let events of small magnitude lull you into complacence about their importance for our physical and mental health.

What might appear to the average person as just a simple daily event may in fact not be so easily overlooked. Its consequences may be much more than just routine outcomes particularly if you cannot make it happen or if you cannot prevent it from happening. Having a shoelace break or a car battery go dead can seriously disrupt your day; in that sense a "simple thing" can turn out to be a threat to your sense of mastery. For example, the weather totally surrounds us and controls us, so much that we do not think of it as a "thing." We are like fish in the proverbial ocean: We do not see the water, but obviously that water has a great deal of influence on how we get through the day.

Of course, you would automatically be aware of major undesirable events such as natural disasters, sudden illness or accidents (such as Jeff Lewis experienced), and other rare but tragic uncontrollable events force us to make major a major shift in our daily habits and routines. On the other hand, someone may give you an unexpected compliment or you may find something uplifting or especially rewarding; a beautiful sunset can be a wonderfully moving experience. But smaller and more routine desirable and undesirable events are certainly more prevalent and perhaps equally influential in our well-being. But in both positive and negative cases, in this Template we are presenting categories of events that are beyond our personal control. Being aware of them and understanding that you cannot control their occurrence is a major step to being able to deal effectively with them. Template #1 is designed to incorporate all possible classes of events which occur outside of your control, be they undesirable, neutral, or desirable, and are of any particular magnitude.

Template #2: Categories of Events That Are Under Your Personal Control

The second major theme of the Serenity Prayer deals with "...grant me the courage to change the things I can." Calling for courage to deal with changeable "things" (we would say "events") may sometimes be necessary, but it seems unlikely that most people need courage to do the things they want to do, while other events may take some extra effort, as implied by the word "courage." I do not want to be too literal in interpreting the Serenity Prayer, but it does give us an inroad into the realm of events that are under our personal control. Under normal circumstances, the category of events under our control subsume desirable events, but sometimes we are personally responsible for undesirable events as well.

As I discussed earlier in Chapter 5 (discussing desirable events), you will recall that I noted how there seemed to be an almost automatic connection between our causing an event to occur and its desirability. Although we sometimes make a mistake and cause ourselves to have an unpleasant experience, in general our lives are filled with occasions when we exercise our personal mastery and achieve a desirable outcome. The question becomes, though, is any given event desirable in and of itself, or do we value it highly because we exercised our personal control to bring it about? Exercising our personal control gives us a boost to our well-being *in principle*, even for routine, small events. The question of the desirability/causation connection becomes important when you realize that we also experience a reasonably high number of desirable experiences caused by someone or something else, without our active causation. A pleasant spring day, hearing a funny story told to us by someone else, or getting a compliment all raise our general well-being even without our own personal causation. Now these experiences fit within our Template #2, that being the general category of events that we experience by asserting our personal mastery to bring them about. Figures 8.1 and 8.2 coming later in this chapter will show you some useful examples of these types of events.

Applying These Templates to Three Categories of Daily Events

The events of the average person's ordinary daily living seem to fall naturally into three main domains or categories of experiences. These are face-valid, and each collects many and varied experiences into a grouping which can cover most if not all of the event experiences a person would normally encounter, some more frequently than others. In each category I have listed major classes of events, and within each class, you can then see how the two Templates of personal causation apply in your life: Either you do or do not have personal control within that class of events.

Your Natural World, the physical environment in which you live. This category groups events in the natural physical environment of everyone on this planet. As you will see, some of these events are controllable by you, some are not.

Your Social World, the world of organized social actions involving you and all other people. This grouping surveys human social groupings, social interactions, social organizations and many forms of social entities that humans have arranged to help themselves and their societies operate efficiently. Again, some of those are outside of your control while you can have controlling effects on others.

Properties of Your World	Not Within Your Control	Within Your Control

Your Natural World	• Natural Disasters
	  • Earthquakes, Floods, Drought, Avalanches
	• Seasonal Cycles
	• Temperature (esp. extremes)
		• Exploring your natural environment
		  • Camping, hiking, swimming, spelunking, travel
		• Hobbies
		  • Photography, astronomy, gardening – farming, gambling
		• Science
		  • Understanding and engineering, predicting, experimenting

Your Social World	• Political World
	  • Laws and governmental:
	    • Rules and regulations
	      • Taxes, fees, licenses, jury duty
	  • Traffic regulations
	    • Signals, lane markers
	  • Police and military regulations
	• Social World
	  • Accidents, crimes
	  • Inducements to actions
	    • Pay, gifts, favors, social approval
	• Economic World
	  • Depressions, recessions, foreclosures, unemployment
		• Organized social activities
		  • Church, school, work, team sports, parties
		• Social connections (ties)
		  • Promises, obligations
		  • Volunteer activities
		• Family activities
		  • Parenting, care giving
		• Giving SRE/ORE
		• Getting married/divorced
		• Engaging in civic activities

Your Personal World	• Childhood experiences
	  • Genetic Endowment
	  • Parental Environment
	    • Nurturing, Supportive
	    • Abusive and neglect
	• Health conditions
	  • Chronic illness
	  • Addictions
	  • Handicaps, disabilities
	• Social experiences
	  • Discrimination, exclusion
	    • Ethnic, religious, political
	• Economic experiences
	  • Poverty, wealth
	  • Work enrichment, difficulty
	  • Job requirements, layoffs
	  • Gambling, outcomes
	    • Lottery winning/losses
	    • Windfall
	  • Cost of living raises
	  • Unemployment compensation
	• School demands (attendance, assignments)
		• Health experiences
		  • Nutrition, diet, exercise
		  • Sports activities
		  • Rehabilitation
		• Intellectual experiences
		  • Extra schooling
		  • Reading workshops
		  • Advanced schooling
		• Entertainment
		  • TV, radio, movies, plays, puzzles
		• Hobbies
		• Volunteer activities

Table 8.1 Listing Examples of The Two Templates for Uncontrollable and Controllable Events For The Three Categories of Daily Events

Your Personal World, the events which you experience as an individual person. At this level, there is the world of events inside your own personal sphere where you most intimately live and have the experience of your own unique events. But as you know by now, there are two classes of events that occur to you as an individual person, some of which you can control, and others you cannot control.

I have combined all of these categories and distinctions into one table that displays how they relate to each other. It is presented in Figure 8.1 opposite.

The Natural Environment:
Template #1: Events Not Under Your Control

Since literally everything under the sun is included in this grouping, some subcategorizing will help to highlight the main differences among the many natural events we can experience in this grouping. Two categories account for these events: They are all just physical entities, responding to physical and chemical laws, but they fall naturally into the hard, physical environment itself, which is populated with inanimate entities and animate, living entities which result from organic processes. Both populate our natural environment, but they fit into our first grouping here because they are all outside of your personal control.

I include here all physical elements of our natural environment, including the asteroids, comets, stars, our sun and moon, the planets, and the universe itself in which our planet the earth has its existence. Not one of these is under our control. But we do spend much time, money, and effort to explore them, to try to understand them (cognitive and interpretive control) and to make predictions about their activities. On our planet, the earth's soil, its mountains, plains, lakes and rivers, and the very atmosphere we breathe, are the physical and organic foundations of our lives. With no personal control over them, we passively endure the processes and events that they cause, such as landslides, earthquakes, tsunamis, volcanic eruptions, hurricanes, tornadoes, floods, and fires and drought. These generally are not caused by humans, at least deliberately. But they can and do intrude on us in desirable and undesirable ways. When undesirable, we become terribly aware of what it is like to have no personal control over these disasters and we can only work to recover from their consequences. But humans do focus many efforts to restore personal control to people who have the misfortune to experience these terrible events. In the wake of the Sumatran tsunami disaster, I suggested to disaster planning and management specialists that they should consider interventions to help people regain a sense of personal control along with the physical survival supplies that they traditionally provide when disasters strike.[3]

Of course, some of these events are not all undesirable: Sunrises and sunsets are often awe-inspiring. Weather changes linked to seasonal cycles often bring us delights such as the wonders of spring and fall. We often change our plans to take advantage of these positive events, and plan around disruptions when the seasons change toward the more unpleasant. For such occurrences as seasons and weather shifts, we automatically employ our accommodation and adaptive control, making ourselves adapt to environments that we cannot make adapt to our own desires. This is "secondary control" as Rothbaum, Weisz, and Snyder describe[4] which I discussed in Chapters 2 and throughout this book, although most researchers do not think of it as secondary.

But uncontrollability is often a problem for us. And our behavior becomes dramatically altered when weather sometimes becomes so completely out of our control that we find that we have difficulty accommodating ourselves to it. Psychologists have studied the effect of hot temperatures on our behaviors finding effects in social disruptions such as riots. Robert

Baron and Virginia Ransberger[5] have studied the occurrence of riots and have found that they are more likely to occur in hot, sweltering temperatures. Craig Anderson, Brad Bushman, and Ralph Groom[6] have shown that other forms of antisocial behavior such as homicide, deadly assault, and rape are also significantly more likely during periods of high temperatures. Interestingly, that relationship does not appear for property crimes such as burglary; apparently these crimes are not related to temperature, suggesting that it is attacking and intending to harm another person that is increased by aversively-hot temperatures.

Of course we humans have not succeeded by being passive recipients of forces beyond our control; we have made ourselves adaptable by trying to accommodate ourselves to these superior forces. This often can pay off nicely. We swim, camp, hike, spelunk, photograph and videotape our environment and travel to exotic ones to explore and enjoy them. Our astronomical telescopes, temperature and humidity and wind speed gauges, space satellites and earthquake predicting instruments all are passive accommodations we have created which give us some predictability of environments we cannot change. These are assertions of our personal mastery. Note, though, that we do not think of them as attempts to change or alter our environments, just to fit in with them. In fact, we pass legislation to set aside parts of our environment which we do not allow ourselves to alter. As demonstrated by our national parks, for instance, we willingly give up control so that the environment is allowed to function and change on its own without our interference.

The other main category of natural events involves living things. In this category I am grouping events which are not under our personal control. We are surrounded by life in its many forms, and they exert favorable and unfavorable effects on us. Starting with the smallest life forms, bacteria have both positive and negative consequences for us. They enable us to get nutrition from plants and animal that we ingest but they can poison us as well. Viruses have stressful if not life-threatening consequences, especially if they mutate into cancer.

On a larger scale, plants provide edible foods, and sustain other life forms such as fish and fowl as part of the global food chain. Forest and grasslands are vast engines of carbon dioxide sequestration, helping to clean the air we breathe. Rivers, lakes, seas and oceans evaporate out moisture which is returned in the form of clouds and rain, having organic consequences. They provide nurturing environments for the myriad of ocean life forms from the smallest krill to the giant whales. We as individuals and as the human race do not cause these to occur.

Of course, we spend a good deal of our lives trying to control the living world. This takes the form of exploiting it, harvesting plant and animal life for our own survival and pleasure. Our control attempts are secondary, in the language of Rothbaum, Weisz, and Snyder, in that we try to adapt and accommodate ourselves to this world with whatever resources we can find available. When we cannot control them and bring them into line with our desires, we do our best by adjusting ourselves by accommodation and acceptance. But these entities, inanimate and living, were present before humans came on the scene. If we humans were to completely leave this early scene, they still will continue in their existence.

The Natural Environment:
Template #2: Events That Are Under Your Control

Humans are resilient, and we show that by the enormous effort we expend to find ways to assert control over our environment of events to make them yield to our needs and desires. Looked at broadly across human history, you can see the major institutions that we created which reflects our aim of engineering our physical environments to make them more acceptable to us. Indeed, the scientific professions of physics, chemistry, biology, medicine, and the engineering and manufacturing professions can be thought of as forms of asserting our control over our environment as much as we can. We farm the land and fish the oceans to acquire our food, build homes to accommodate to weather extremes, and we build dams to mitigate drought and to grow our crops. We use our chemistry and biology to create new clothes and new foods, often creating things that do not exist in the natural world. We train physicians to control the impact of diseases, and we build hospitals and clinics where, in those unnatural environments, we try to gain control over pathogens which can harm us if they are not controlled, at least to some degree.

We build planes, trains, and automobiles to conquer distance. We make artificial materials that keep us warmer or cooler than nature creates. We burn coal, oil, and natural gas to create heat to keep us comfortable and productive, and we chill the air for our homes, factories, and movie theaters. We build giant covered stadiums so that we can control our climate as we watch, vicariously, our favorite sports heroes try to defeat their opponents (obscuring, perhaps, that we have no personal control over the action). In our homes, we make electrons jump to our command to turn our appliances (which we created) off and on, and we artificially split atoms to make them yield up their power to run those appliances. We cannot control lightning, but Benjamin Franklin found out how it works and Thomas Edison and Nicola Tesla and Charles Steinmetz learned how to generate it artificially and use it to control our world.

These controlling actions are so common that we are mostly unaware of them. We are the planet's most effective personal control machines. Still, though, there is the world of uncontrollable events, and at some very fundamental level, everything could turn against us. Forces on this planet, and outside of us, are so powerful that we could become completely overwhelmed and could lose all of our control, and perhaps our lives in the process. This possibility suggests that we should always be realistic in our thoughts about our real power in the environment in which we find ourselves.

Summary: Highlights of this Section

Although we are not always conscious of our physical and natural environment, it would do us well to think of it in terms of the personal mastery perspective. We can strengthen our beliefs in our ability to get the goals we desire and avoid negative experiences if we think of ourselves as enmeshed in a physical environment. We gain personal mastery by engaging in pleasurable activities such as the many forms of outdoor recreation (hiking, biking, swimming, exploring, etc.) as these are directly under our personal control. I deliberately mention these activities because they are non-social; they do not have to include other people. I have reserved events in our social environment for the next main section of this chapter.

In short, our physical environment offers us a world of desirable experiences. We are usually fully aware of them and we are happy to take the initiative and make our personal choices to engage in them. There is a double bang-for-the-buck here: The events are desirable in and of themselves, and choosing to engage in them is an assertion of our personal mastery motivations.

But in many cases, sometimes the environment is out of our control and contains threats, risks, and dangers to our well-being. But our two-fold approach to control again shows us a way to gain from this class of experiences: Not only are you able to pursue desirable events, also you can make efforts to avoid undesirable events. In the case of your physical environment, this means exerting diligence and foresight to prevent threatening events from taking place at all, having adequate physical and financial resources to stop things from happening. We can gain positive feelings about ourselves by "being prepared" in the language of Boy Scouts. Even more, though, should undesirable physical events "happen" to you, you have a range of choices to accommodate yourself to the particular properties of the (uncontrollable) events, as described by Rothbaum, Weisz, and Snyder. Rather than trying to change the situation, you can control your personal reactions and adapt by finding alternative paths to take, make substitutions for your adaptation, and you can take precautions to prevent a recurrence of the event. You can ultimately acknowledge that you have no power to alter the unalterable, should that be necessary, and take comfort in your ability to "live with it." That is the main message of the Serenity Prayer. This choice is a form of personal control. This ultimate withdrawal need not be thought of as a defeat, but as a smart move under otherwise uncontrollable circumstances. Some people take comfort in believing that "it is God's will" and accept that as an understandable and acceptable way to guide their lives.

The Social Environment:
Template #1: Events That Are Not Under Your Control

At the instant of your birth you are surrounded by a social environment of doctors and nurses and mothers and fathers and family. Your social world is just as enveloping as your natural world. We give over control over large chunks of our life to social events and other people, so in this sense we live much of our lives literally, "out of control" (as I use the concept in this book). This is an important point to make when you think of personal mastery in your life. I want to describe that situation in this section, and in the next section I will describe the multitude of ways which in fact we do assert control over our social environment, even though, again, we may not be consciously aware of it.

For whatever historical reasons and by whatever historical mechanisms, very early on we humans banded together to live in social units: We created families, tribes, and nations out of this near-universal tendency. In these developments, people established expectations for desirable and undesirable behavior and developed ways to enforce those expectations. Sociologists and social psychologists explain these enforced regularities in social behavior as reflections of "norms," which David Myers[7] has neatly defined as, "...the rules for expected and accepted behavior" (p. 120). Norms have evolved over the centuries and get transmitted to the infant through parental encouragement and explicit training. Out of these traditions we have evolved legal entities called laws. These are initially external to the individual, and you as an individual have no personal control over the presence or the enforcement of these expectations and standards of behavior (laws). Indeed, it is thought that the internalization of external norms into the individual's own personal conscious life is a major factor in the socialization process.

This is the complex, long-term process whereby the individual becomes an integrated member of the family unit and, more generally, a functional member of society. Failure to follow the norms leads to sanctions and punishments imposed either informally by social disapproval or formally by legally-empowered authorities. Law itself can be described as a set of socially-agreed upon formal rules for controlling the behavior of the individual. In this sense, control is totally external to the individual person, deliberately so. Perhaps the most controlling of all social entities is the military. Obedience is taught from day one, and maintained by a rigid top-down structure in which deviations from discipline are strictly sanctioned. On the other hand, military units can be marvelously effective in achieving goals necessary to the survival of the unit, and the nation.

History is filled with individuals and groups who choose to assert their personal control by violating the external standards. It is called nonconformity and law-breaking for the individual, and rebellion, war, and revolution in the case of groups.

Depending on whose side you are on, this rejection of external standards is either heretical or heroic. When these efforts succeed, they are called revolutionary heroes; otherwise, they are called rebels. In either case, the personal mastery perspective provides us a model for understanding the psychology of the individual person surrounded by an uncontrollable social environment. To describe this section, there are many ways of categorizing the classes of social events which exist independent of the individual and outside of his/her control. I will start out with the largest and most inclusive, then move toward classes of events which are likely to be more directly visible to you as an individual in your society as you go about the activities of your daily living.

Laws: Government and Organizational Rules and Regulations. In theory, everyone is subject to the laws of their country. There are many structures, processes and set procedures which sustain that society as a going entity. We are obligated to sit on a jury when called. We are obligated to pay taxes on our property and our incomes. We are required to pay various fees for services, licenses, registration costs, and other charges for the benefits we derive from using those services. Governments regulate our behavior in the form of traffic laws, speed limits, driving lanes, and the active presence of police to enforce them. They are empowered to take away some of our personal control if we violate the rules. They can control us with speeding and parking tickets and, for more serious violations, jail time. These external constraints are so pervasive that most people grow up with them and obey them automatically without directly experiencing those painful sanctions, but knowing full well that these are ever-present and to be avoided.

Naturally no one enjoys having to give up some of their freedom to act as they choose. This issue of giving up our freedom or resisting external controlling pressure has received considerable research attention by psychologists. The most direct investigation of this situation was initiated by Jack Brehm and his colleagues.[8] They theorized that people have a deep-lying tendency to react against threats to their freedom of choice and action. A state of "psychological reactance" arises when an external force threatens to take away the person's freedom. A common reaction is to reassert the threatened freedom of action. In fact, you can undermine a person's belief in something if you tell them that (in the wording of one of their investigations of this issue), "You have no choice but to believe this."[9] Some people go faster when they see a speed limit sign, or will trespass on private property when seeing a posted sign saying "Keep Out." Children will spread more litter at a swimming pool area when they see a sign that says, "Don't Litter."[10] From a personal control perspective, this fighting back against external pressures is one obvious key to why social control is often a problem in modern societies.

Economic Forces. Modern societies function by establishing economic structures, policies, and procedures which give us agreed-upon standards of procedure involving our finances. The structures are maintained by sanctions for violations. Those sanctions are impersonal; they are not under an individual's personal control, and an individual's freely chosen actions have to occur within a constricted range of choices. You cannot print your own money, and you have to be sure that the money other people give you fits the approved standards. It is to the advantage of individuals to accommodate themselves to the system. We learn to take advantage of the exchange of goods and services. This accommodation gives each person predictable ways to engage in organized economic interactions with other people. We buy their services, and they buy ours, with all parties understanding the ways that economic exchanges work. That is the desirable side of economic arrangements. The undesirable side is when things go wrong, such as recessions, depressions, and inflation which wreck our accepted arrangements.

Sometimes the frustration of facing an uncontrollable economic world results in serious social discontent. Joseph Hepworth and Stephen West[11] confirmed earlier research suggesting that there was a consistent relationship between the occurrence of lynching of black men and cotton prices in the American South between 1882 and 1930. As cotton prices and the value of cotton land slumped during hard times, the frequency of the lynching of black men increased, an indication of a relationship between frustration and aggression in the sphere of economics.

At a more personal level, we can find jobs available to us in good times and unavailable in bad times, but in both times we have no individual personal control over the larger social/economic forces that create and destroy jobs. But we can find ways to accommodate ourselves to these forces by developing skills and experiences that can get us a job with pay; with that income, we gain some freedom of choice and greater personal mastery. But we personally can be effective only with limits, and all of us are always in danger of being swept aside by uncontrollable economic forces. As I write this, the American people are only now seeing a reduction in bankruptcies, home foreclosures, and high levels of unemployment due to rampant speculation in the era of the early-2000s. It is a relief to see better times ahead, but no one single individual has the controlling power to bring them about.

Social Organizations and Entities. Societies are woven from the creation, compounding and integration of formal and informal social structures. These structures evolve and become relatively stable or even rigid as they take over control of individuals. Almost any organization can be thought of as such an entity. Most likely you will find yourself to be a "member" in some way of at least one or more of those entities. I can only briefly touch on some of the more prominent ones functioning today.

The Military. Perhaps the most structured of all organizations in any society is the military. Organized for the purpose of protecting and maintaining the larger society, this entity systematically reduces the personal control of any individual and moves all control up the structure to the top ranks. Obedience and giving up one's personal control is required. Individual initiative is possible, but it is usually highly constrained and is unlikely to change the external organizational structure itself.

Business Organizations. Similar to the military, businesses are organized to achieve financial goals with a minimum of organizational disruption by its employees. This requires considerable normative control over individuals, although flexibility and initiative often are rewarded. Sometimes it is necessary to restructure the organization but there is a resistance and inertia to maintain the structure as long as it is achieving goals successfully. Individuals are expected to conform to the structure's norms by yielding to the control asserted by the management.

Church and Religious/Spiritual Organizations. Some religious organizations such as the Catholic Church are highly structured and place considerable external control over the religious beliefs and activities of the individual. Within other religious organizations considerably more flexibility in church organization and individual initiative is more common. Nevertheless, the norms of the organization are inculcated in the individual, usually at an early age, and adherence to the norms is maintained by a strong network of social relations among church members.

Political Parties. Even more loosely organized than religious institutions but still built around a core of political and economic beliefs, political parties find it important to create some strong structure and organizational principles to be able to function effectively and to win votes. Individual adherence is necessary at the higher levels of the organization, with lessening strictures at the lower levels. Even at that, though, personal identification with the party's norms is expected, and to that extent personal choice is reduced and compliance with the ongoing activities and principles of the party is expected.

The Social Environment:
Template #2: Events That Are Under Your Control

While we live in the social world with its organizations and systems of norms that constrain our own freedom of action, we are also nested within a network of socially-based actions which we create for ourselves by exercising our own free will. To a considerable degree, we create our own social environments and interact with other people in ways that we personally choose. Once beyond infancy and childhood, we start to be more capable of getting what we want within our social environment. The choices we make often involve our connections and bonds with other people. Interestingly, we often freely give up our freedom of choice by making commitments, obligations and promises to others. In this section I discuss those obligations which directly involve other people; in a later section I will discuss those which are more individualistic and do not intentionally involve other people. I begin this discussion here with a focus on our intimate social relations and then move to larger-scale social activities.

Marriage and Divorce. Getting married, at least in many cultures, is a freely-chosen action. As such, it brings with it an entire realm of events and experiences to which we commit ourselves, asserting our personal control. Interestingly, not all of our experiences end up being entirely self-chosen; marriage engages sharing and giving up our own desires to help our partner achieve their desires. This giving up part of our freedom of choice is a form of accommodation by changing the self. But when we make that accommodation, that nevertheless resides on a foundation of free-choice and personal commitment. But sometimes things can go wrong, and separation and divorce result from the strictures and loss of our freedom of action inherent in these arrangements. Free choice may be more difficult to locate in this complicated circumstance, but ultimately some form of accommodation and choice about how to function are engaged in our personal resolution of marital problems.

Family Relations, Parenting and Caregiving. Marriage often leads to children and with that comes the activities deeply imbedded in child care. Even without children, though, we have our parents and other family members which creates enduring obligations and ties; we become immersed in a life filled with events and activities involved in maintaining those social relations. These can be times of great happiness and self-actualization. Sometimes illness and accidents can intrude in the lifestyles and these external causes force us to change and to make accommodations in the way we handle them (adjustment, in the sense of secondary control). Control over the other person is a key part of this. When family members need our aid, we can encourage them to be self-reliant (SRE: see the discussion of my research on this in Chapter 2[12,13]) or we can encourage them to rely on us to help them, (ORE: Other–reliance encouragement). The choices we make about how to "help" another person reflect the personal choices we make to accommodate ourselves to those social relationships which in effect reside outside of our sphere of control.

Social Connections and Ties Outside of Marriage and Family. Our growth as an adult follows a path from the narrow confines of the family into outer circles of ever-expanding social connections. Those social connections engage our desires and choices, but they also engage promises, obligations, and expectations of others. Our success at enjoying our social living is determined by how we balance our sense of free choice with our ability to accommodate ourselves to the desires and expectations that others have of us. My colleague Robert Cialdini[14] has explored these subtle connections, noting that key components of successful interpersonal influence involves reciprocity, the ordinary give-and-take in which people do favors for one another. In this sense, we give up some of our "pure" freedom by accepting, implicitly or explicitly, the obligation to return the favor. In most norm-based interactions, everyone falls into these patterns without losing their beliefs in their own personal mastery. But the "system" can become polluted when scam artists manipulate us for their own illicit gain. It is called fraud, and nothing is more punishing to our sense of mastery and control in our lives when we find out that our trust in the system has been violated. The financial loss hurts, but equally painful is the loss of interpersonal trust; it is a signal that your life has gotten out of control.

Summary: Highlights of this Section

The personal mastery approach provides a unique and productive way of thinking of our lives as surrounded by our physical environment, as I just discussed. That way of thinking provides a natural fit with another key aspect of our lives, our *social* environment. And following the model suggested in the two templates, there are two distinct facets of our social life; the realm of events we can control, and the realm of events we cannot control. I want to extract some highlights of this discussion of the various classes of social events in our lives.

There are many ways in which we control our own social behavior, meshing our own personal mastery beliefs and actions in light of our social relationships. To a very real extent, our own life is strongly colored by how we treat others, and they treat us. The personal mastery perspective reveals a number of subtle but important ways in which our exercise of our control in dealing with others can greatly enhance our own life satisfaction and well-being. The downside is a loss to some degree of personal control, but adjustment and accommodation to the needs and wishes of others helps build strong and enduring social bonds for the benefit of all.

On the other hand, our freedom of choice is at least reduced or even controlled by our social environment. It exerts control over us by the enforcement effects of external sanctions, varying from "soft norms" which we internalize and accept as our own personal norms to social forces which exert great pressure to conform. We resist these at some peril to our well-being. But we still have available to us the choice of accommodation. It is much more than just "giving up." We are armed with a powerful set of capacities for adjusting to superior forces in our life, and good adjustment and resilience in the face of stronger forces can be linked with successful secondary control actions. Of course, if the "person/environment fit" (PXE) is not a good one, you can end up with discontent, deviations, and sometimes even breaking of the law and disobedience to the norms of the organization. This also highlights one difference between the natural world and the social world: The natural world alters and changes by the operation of its own forces, whereas in the social world changes occur when enough individuals choose to deviate and try to change the way their organization functions. This is where revolutions begin, by choice.

Your Own Personal World:
Template #2: Events That Are Not Under Your Control

The next two sections now will focus on your own "personal environment," your world of events, of personal experiences in your own "life space." This is not to claim that the natural world and the social world are totally outside of your own personal life; they are inevitably a part of how you live. But the personal mastery perspective suggests that there is a myriad of events and experiences that occur within a narrow range that is specific to just you, as a single individual. This is the world of "mine," of "my," of "belongs to me." They are unique to your own experiences and they are not necessarily shared with anyone else. And as I did in the above sections, I will separate out two classes of your personal experiences, those that occur from outside your own personal causation, and those that you yourself cause to occur. First will be your events which are outside of your personal control.

Birth and Early Childhood. Although this may perhaps sound a bit scary or harsh, when you were born into your life you were dominated by forces completely outside of your control: You are born as a helpless (literally) infant, surrounded by your mother, physicians, nurses, perhaps your father, and assorted other clinical personnel. But you did not choose to have any of the experiences that happened to you. Naturally you were not given any control over the genetic and biological processes which came with your conception and birth. These forces controlled and regulated your biochemical and neuromuscular reactions to the world as they impinged on your innate sensory capacities. All of these endowments have played a crucial and a continuing role in your physical survival and your well-being throughout life. So you began your life with no personal control, surviving only through dependence on your physical and social environment.

Given this helplessness, it is important that you be given an adaptive, functioning genetic endowment and a nurturing, supportive, and growth-enhancing social environment (here is the PXE model again). These are the foundations from which a sense of personal mastery may arise. They are the most common child rearing conditions, fortunately for society. But, unfortunately, abuse and neglect of infants and children do happen, so social control can be malevolent, leading to long-term problems for children who are exposed to such conditions. Penelope Trickett and Catherine McBride-Chang[15] conducted an extensive review of the research literature on the effects of abusive earlychildhood environments. Here is a quotation from one of their major conclusions derived from their review:

...there is no longer any doubt that maltreatment – whether it be sexual abuse, physical abuse, neglect, or some mixture – has significant adverse effects on the development and adjustment of children, adolescents, and adults (p. 324).

Social Experiences Beyond Childhood. Since you had no control over your genetics or your social environment at your birth, you also were not given any control over your bodily health and well-being. Some babies are "born beautiful," and research shows that attractive babies receive more attention and favorable treatment from their parents than less attractive ones.[16] That favorable treatment continues throughout life, even though the person has little or no control over it. Studies on what researchers call the "what-is-beautiful-is-good" stereotype[17,18] show that more attractive people are thought by other people to have a better character. Beautiful people are perceived to be more honest, more trustworthy, and more competent; they receive more votes when running for office, lesser penalties for misdemeanors, and of course they are top draws for media and television productions. You should be so lucky. But it is not initially in your control to be beautiful; you were born that way. Billions of dollars are spent annually by people seeking to attain more beauty. From a personal mastery control point of view, of course, this could be a losing proposition, in the sense that you are placing your self-worth in the hands of others. Some people make millions off their appearance, but when they can no longer keep up their beauty, we have to wonder what has happened to their sense of personal mastery in the process of losing that nice appearance.

There is a more directly unfortunate side of this external control. Stereotyping, prejudice, and discrimination are often based on personal characteristics over which the person has no personal control. People born with the "wrong" skin color, the wrong body shape or deformity or even the "wrong" sex, are subjected to external social sanctions such as differential and negative treatment, discrimination and exclusion from the majority of society's desirable activities. You are given ethnic, religious, economic status at birth, yet receive favorable or unfavorable treatment as if you had something to do with it.

In other areas of life, health conditions that we experience are often outside of our control, both in infancy and throughout our lifetime. I discussed the relationship between personal mastery and our health in earlier chapters, but how people regard us and actually treat us because of the state of our health that we are "given" is not under our own personal control. Handicaps, chronic illness, and disabilities are often met with some form of social withdrawal by others, reflecting a tendency to stigmatize those who are different, a point made earlier in a classic work by Erving Goffman.[19] When politics, religion, and preferences and personal tastes get brought into the picture of how we relate to others, then there is an almost infinite number of ways we can be stigmatized and rejected by others. Being "different" is to a large extent out of your control. Facing that, we still have available to us many alternative ways of coping with the reactions of others. People find ways to cope with social exclusion but their adjustment is likely to be relatively unsatisfactory unless they can see that coping as an assertion of their personal mastery. You can maintain your belief in your own personal mastery by controlling your own reactions, even if you cannot control theirs.

Economic Events Beyond Your Control. Modern societies run on the basis of their economic system and the individual person has little control over how it functions or malfunctions. The world of external economic forces has its consequences inside our own personal world. Recessions and depressions arise and force changes on the individual. You can be laid off or fired for reasons beyond your control. You can reassert your control by choosing to seek another job, or train for a different or better one. But even with a job, requirements of the position are set by higher-ups outside of your own choices. Your cost of living is only partly controllable by you, but inflation or deflation or, worse, economic depression, can undermine your best efforts. On the positive side of this, government can set the minimum wage level, it can provide cost of living raises, and unemployment compensation provides a safety net under almost everyone. Social security benefits are available in most advanced societies and the healthcare system provides a platform for maintenance of your health. In terms of financial security and advancement, this range of external controlling events has been created by society to help you keep engaged in pursuing your own welfare.

In the next section, I will describe the other half of your personal world and how you come to manage the events of your life when you are able to personally control them.

Your Own Personal World:
Template #2: Events That Are Under Your Control

This Template will strike you as dealing with the most common and familiar part of your life. After all, we get along in life by bringing it within our realm of personal control, so that we can achieve our aims and move forward in life. You can think about your personally controllable events consisting of two classes of occurrences: (1) exercising your personal mastery to cause desirable events, and (2) exercising your personal mastery to prevent undesirable events from occurring. As you can tell from all that has gone before, this section applies very usefully to your physical and your mental health. You should think of this section as an introduction and overview to the next chapter, my final chapter, in which I will present the personal mastery experiment that my colleagues and I developed to enhance the personal mastery experience of our research participants. That experiment ties together all of the strands that make up the core of this treatment of personal mastery concepts in this book.

Applying Template #2 to Your Health and Well-Being: Your Physical Health

How to Achieve Your Desirable Events

Your Body and Your Physical Health: We can begin this section at the most basic level, the physical entity of your body. I just described in the previous section your birth as an event which is out of your control. But we all grow up, and life can be seen from a personal mastery perspective as a process in which you gain increasing control over the events in your life. So once you are born and functioning independently, your interactions with your world then become completely different. Surely your physical body is the most controllable aspect of your life. Given average health, we can think of your body as the machine which carries out your wishes, goals, and the plans you personally develop to carry them out. There are many ways in which you control events that relate to your physical body and these get quickly reflected in your well-being.

Increase Your Physical Assets: Your body is your temple, and you are primarily responsible for keeping it healthy and growing. We now know that good nutrition and routine exercise are keys to bodily health, and both are fully under your own personal control. Many people feel that good appearance is highly important, so good grooming can benefit your mental health; billions of dollars are spent annually as people assert their control in exactly this way. I would caution, though, that activity is health-supporting, as long as people do it for their self-improvement and not to please other people; that would amount to allowing there to be an external determinant of one's actions.

Beyond our childhood we develop better personal control over our basic biological processes. Toilet training is perhaps our first introduction to personal control, but all forms of restraint, suspension of immediate drives and postponing need gratification are extensions of this control into later stages of maturity. There are training and exercise regimens such as yoga and meditation which you can use to lower your oxygen uptake and your heart rate; learning to use them can bring your blood pressure to more healthful levels. Those techniques are "mental" in the sense that the person performs the exercises without needing artificial external causes. Such external causes as medications and biofeedback equipment can change a number of bodily conditions but at some level it is up to the individual to make the choice to use them. The mastery perspective would argue that there is risk for dependence on such artificial external causes; addiction and serious loss of control can result from extended uses of drugs and other forms of external causes.

How to Avoid Undesirable Physical Events: As I discussed in the earlier chapters, poor health is a major factor in decreasing beliefs in one's personal mastery. It can lead to depression and anxiety as well as stresses in our social life. Prevention of poor health should be a top consideration for anyone. This requires ongoing attention to cleanliness and high levels of personal hygiene. Routine medical check-ups are helpful to monitor the state of your resistance to infections and your vital signs. Promptly seeking medical advice and, if necessary, treatment at the first signs of potential problems will help control the problems, perhaps prevent them, and ameliorate symptoms should they occur. The normal reduction of capacity with aging is to be expected but good health and an active lifestyle have been shown in countless studies to be the best offense against the threats of older age.

Applying Template #2 to Your Health and Well-Being: Your Mental Health

How to Achieve Your Desirable Events
The central dimensions of your mental health revolve around intellectual, cognitive, and emotional achievements. Education

and studying to improve your mental skills and your cognitive sharpness are easily available to you in public and private educational opportunities, including almost numberless online choices. Life-long learning is now a cultural norm, and re-tooling is now necessary in almost all vocational activities. Hobbies such as art, music, writing, and sports and outdoor activities, volunteering to help others are all easily available and can readily be integrated into an active, vibrant lifestyle. Your mental health can be sustained through religious and spiritual commitments and activities and through life-long opportunities for engaging in personally-chosen ways of engaging with the many forms of organized and informal religious organizations. These are your own beliefs, and developing and sustaining them throughout life is central to your beliefs in your mastery of your own life.

How to Decrease Your Undesirable Events.

There are many threats to our mental health in our daily living above and beyond our physical life. Depression and anxiety are major national concerns. Insecurity, stress, uncertainty and unpreparedness for unexpected events are always present in modern life. The best antidote is to avoid uncontrollable stresses such as financial downturns, losses of jobs, friends or even loved ones, and to develop as early as possible adequate financial and educational and social networks so that you have available a reserve of assets providing you with resources for facing possible losses. Taking on unsupportable financial commitments (credit card debt, loans to others, unwise borrowing or financial investments, *etc.*) are heavy stressors that can get out of your control. Social losses can be as devastating as financial losses, so developing a broad and deep network of friends and acquaintances is recommended and, of course, this is under your control to a significant degree. Preparedness is under your control, and you can gain a stronger sense of personal mastery if you engage your best resources for resilience.

Summary: Highlights of this Section

As with the two previous major sections of this chapter, I want to summarize this discussion of your personal mastery and control concerning the events in your environment. Again, I will follow our model of interpreting your world from two perspectives: How your actions can increase your desirable events and how you can act to decrease undesirable events.

At our birth, we are placed into a completely uncontrollable world. We have our genetic endowment and native biological functions which are focused on guaranteeing our survival, but we have no developed sense of personal mastery itself. This grows as we grow. And in addition to the physical world, we also have our social world, some of which can help us survive and grow, but some of which does not help. Our physical looks and our state of health, both out of our own control, bring us supportive or harmful events which impinge on us. As we mature, our own distinctive personality and skills set become engage in our pursuit of desirable experiences and our control over threatening events which we strive to avoid. Overall, our mental and physical well-being depends on the success with which our endowments mesh with the world of uncontrollable and controllable events into which we are born. Eventually we move into our own personal sphere of established beliefs, thought, and actions result from gaining greater personal mastery. Our lives become oriented toward developing and enhancing our physical health through such actions as we develop good diet and exercise habits while we avoid unhealthful events and practices. We grow intellectually, developing mental skills and habits of critical thinking along with acquiring job skills and emotional intelligence to engage more effectively with other people.

Making These Distinctions Apply to
Your Actions and Activities

In Figure 8.1 earlier in this chapter I intended to help make you aware of useful distinctions among the almost innumerable types of events that you experience in your own life, distinctions provided by the personal mastery approach. Now it is time to move from awareness to *actions and activities* as you can choose to assert your personal mastery in your daily living. The question arises of applying what you now know about personal mastery to actually doing something about your desires and your demands, your controllable and uncontrollable events, the supporting and challenging events that you experience as you grow throughout your life. Putting your insights and knowledge into action in appropriate and successful ways requires paying attention both to yourself and to the properties of the environment that surround you. This means applying the PXE match model that I have discussed many times throughout this book. That also means, particularly, applying your own personal Template #1 and Template #2 to your daily experiences. I have developed a graphic display of how all of these parts can interrelate with each other, with you and your personal mastery beliefs at the center of how all of these properties of events are interconnected: They are connected through *you* and the choice of actions you can take! Figure 8.2 displays the relationships between you and your environment from the perspective provided by the two Templates.

In the Figure, I have placed at its center your core personal mastery beliefs surrounded by uncontrollable and controllable events grouped as desirable, neutral, and undesirable. The circle filling the box has a solid line. I have used shading and a solid circular line to indicate that there is a barrier of a sort between you and uncontrollable events, while that circular line is dashed to indicate that you are much more open to your world of controllable events. Finally, the wordings around your core personal mastery beliefs indicate that you are free to choose to change yourself when faced with uncontrollable events, while if you choose to exercise your choices, you will be more able to change your world when you want to pursue controllable events.

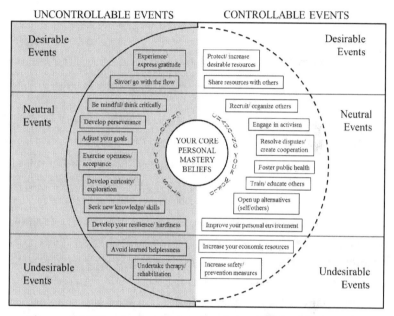

Figure 8.1 Displaying Behavioral Available Choices for Actions in The Personal Mastery Approach to Daily Living.

As you study the Figure, try to add in your own personal actions and activities that match with the properties of any given quadrant. Interestingly, when you do that, you will be in the position of making a response that you think is appropriate for that particular situation. This question ultimately boils down to our *choices*, what particular actions we choose when faced with controllable or uncontrollable events. There are many ways to think about what is really a matter of a PXE fit... how you match your choices of actions with the world in which you find yourself. In Fig. 8.2, I have selected some obvious everyday actions we take in our world, but I have linked those choices with event valence (desirable, neutral, and undesirable) controllability. Within each combination, I have listed some particular types of choices we can and do make. As usual in this book, I am listing generalized examples. As you read over them, you can of course come up with your own particular examples of how you respond when you experience a particular example of a particular class of events. In effect, this picture is a template of the PXE approach that has infused this entire book. This point of intersection is how you can create and apply your own personal control template.

You and Your Personal Control in Your Environment

I have now come full circle in this book. I began this book by presenting the Serenity Prayer. Translated into modern psychological thinking, and especially with attention to the concept of empowerment it seems to imply, I have presented a great amount of research which supports what it means to be empowered: To have a strong sense of personal mastery and a belief that you can be a success at the two main paths of life that the personal mastery suggests: By being successful at achieving desirable goals, and being able to prevent the occurrence in your life of undesirable experiences. The two Templates I developed encapsulate the main theme of the Serenity Prayer, but this book is a wide-ranging review of psychological research and clinical practice that have tested its basic ideas and have repeatedly supported its usefulness. I believe that the results show a high degree of proved support for the Prayer. But now we have a broader and deeper understanding of the basic principles that underlie it. And those principles have the advantage of showing you how to apply specific actions in specific circumstances to assert effectively your chosen actions. And, perhaps equally valuable, they give you useful insights into how other people are dealing with their own personal worlds of controllable and uncontrollable experiences.

Throughout this book I have followed a model of mental health followed by nearly all psychological researchers and therapists: the Person X Environment Model in which the characteristics of the person are best understood by how those characteristics match, or fail to match, the characteristics of the environment. Your sense of personal mastery and ability to control the events of your life do or do not match the controlling properties of your environment. A match is a key to better adjustment and mental health, while a fail to match is a risk factor for lower life satisfaction. You may enhance your "matching" from what you have read in this book.

Applying These Principles in Your Own Life

With these principles and Template in mind, it is now time to see how my colleagues and I developed and experimentally tested an organized program for helping people achieve greater mastery in their daily living. The next chapter presents a tested and successful experimental intervention weaving together many of the ideas I have discussed in this book. If I have convinced you of the power of the personal mastery approach in the many studies I reviewed, then you should easily see the ways in which you can adopt these for creating a new lifestyle for yourself.

Chapter 9

A Proven Personal Mastery Intervention

I have now discussed what research has shown to be the key components for developing a project which you can apply to you own personal mastery beliefs and actions. You have a framework which integrates two key dimensions of the events we experience as we go through life. First, that framework requires specifying the *emotional and evaluative* properties of events: Those that are desirable, those that are undesirable, and the broad and rather unexplored and heterogeneous class of events that are neutral and ordinary. Naturally, the most research attention has been on the first two, but logically the third category is itself of interest because the basic principles of personal causation apply to them as well. Second, that framework also integrates the desirable event/undesirable event property with the processes of *personal causation*: Some events are caused by us, and some are caused by the world outside of us.

We have now come full circle. In this framework, we can see that people spend much of their lives trying to make desirable events occur while also trying to prevent undesirable events from occurring. Research shows the broad-band favorable effects on our mental and physical health the more that we are successful in those attempts. Much of what we have discussed is not just common sense. As I said in the Introduction, the question of trying to be happy is a tricky one, but it is not a trick one. The overall message of the personal mastery approach research leads me to think that pursuing mastery and personal control over the events of your life is likely to be a more productive and satisfying goal of life.

Integrating and cross-connecting the two categories of the control dimension of events with the three evaluative categories of events creates a 3x2 framework or template for you to understand how all of the parts of your personal mastery beliefs and actions fit together. Also, understanding these principles will give you insights into how other people have organized their lives, some successfully, some not so successfully. You can have a clearer insight into how to respond to those people once you see how they perceive events in their lives. Also, we take seriously the results from some of our prior studies. Recall from Chapter 3 my discussion of the study with my colleagues McCall, Grossman, Zautra, and Guarnaccia.[1] We assessed not only whether or not a demand or desire event had occurred but also whether or not the person had responded to the event and, if so, how satisfying the experience had been. We showed that a higher amount of experiencing externally-caused events was related to poorer quality of life; however, when the person engaged in a higher level of actually *dealing* with those events, then that led to a better quality of life. This was particularly the case if the person were feeling more satisfaction with the outcome of that event experience.

The role of actually responding to an event was again supported in our "2 vs. 12" study.[2] When people engage in many positive events (12) as opposed to a few (2) over a two-week period, the 12 group reports higher mental health if they have recently been experiencing a high number of undesirable events, a buffering effect. Overall, then, our studies consistently show the value of actual actions in dealing with daily events, as opposed to passively just experiencing them. Although much of the research literature on personal mastery treats it as a system of beliefs, our research shows that the "action component" is a major factor in its positive effects on our mental health. As you will see later in this chapter, we made it a major component of our experimental test of our personal control intervention.

You will recall that in Chapter 6, I described a number of different therapies and interventions for enhancing personal control. Although all of them proved successful in enhancing some particular aspect of well-being, no one intervention project melded the two key dimensions for control and evaluation into one integrated, systematic project. Consequently, my colleagues Alex Zautra, Mary Davis, and I took on that challenge and developed an integrated experimental intervention to enhance personal mastery. We developed it in a pilot project as a spin-off from a larger project studying the physical and mental health of middle-age adults which we had already gotten underway. Both projects were funded by the National Institute on Aging[3] and a more detailed technical report on the project I am describing in this chapter is published and now available for the public.[4]

First, a Note on Technology

As you read through the personal mastery interventions I discussed in Chapter 6, you will note that all of them are conducted in small groups such as nursing homes, small groups of experimental volunteers, *etc*. Although all of these studies have shown good results, their practical implications are rather limited because up until recently there has been no obvious way to export those techniques to larger groups. Very recently, however, technology has advanced to such an amazing degree that the limitations of practicality in previous studies can be overcome with modern communications systems. I am speaking here of telephone communicability combined with automated calling systems. With these systems, an almost limitless number of people can be contacted *via* their cell phones, and any prerecorded messages can be delivered to them easily and efficiently.

In our study, we were able to employ automated telephone contact and message delivering systems to communicate with our volunteer participants. In turn, they were able with a computerized answer system *via* internet connectivity to return to us their responses to a set of evaluation and assessment questions assessing the usual mental and physical health measures I have discussed in my earlier research reviews. The participants did not have to be in a group nor were they restricted to any particular residential situation. In fact, they usually were at home or work and could be contacted completely independently of any other specific situations. With our technology, we were able to contact them in their "natural environment," going about their daily business. Overall, they could easily receive our communicated messages and could easily implement them in their daily, ongoing lives.

This project was successfully completed and demonstrated, in principle, the value and power of modern communication technology to expand personal mastery manipulations to essentially unlimited numbers of participants and to assess the outcomes continuously and efficiently. That will become clear as I describe the study in the next section: I will present the details on how the project was conducted, followed by highlights of some of the key results. Although the project had many facets, I will keep my focus here only on the Personal Mastery enhancement condition.

Let me give you a quick overview and a context for reading about the study. Our results showed that, compared to a comparison condition that was also part of the study, the Personal Mastery treatment condition resulted in several better mental health outcomes than the comparison condition. You can then see how we developed our ideas into a workable format for presenting them to our participants as they went about their daily living. You may wish to take advantage of this material by adopting it into your own life.

Procedures of the Experimental Intervention

The project began with the recruitment of adults 40-65 years old who were residents of Phoenix, Arizona and surrounding areas who met our initial screening and inclusion criteria: Middle-aged and who scored at least at a moderate level of depressive thoughts and emotions on a quick-form screening test of depression. That was the target population of our larger study. Depression would be of particular interest to us since, as you will recall from my discussion in Chapter 2. Clinical research has shown that there is a reliable connection between feelings of loss of control (or externality) and depression.[5,6]

To locate potential participants, community-residing adults were contacted by telephone and given general information about an experimental project to promote their well-being. The discussion at that point was a general overview and orientation, but the participants also responded to a brief screening inventory to detect the presence of at least moderate feelings of depression. Those people who reported at least some symptoms and agreed to participate were formally enrolled in the study and scheduled for a follow-up in-person meeting with our project staff.

At that meeting, those who agreed to continue with us were given a set of "pre" questionnaires assessing a wide range of standard physical and mental health measures of wide use in psychological research. The very same questions were again answered at the end of the project approximately a month later in a "post" questionnaire. Testing for pre-post differences provided a strong test of any effects of the intervention (again, compared to the comparison group sample, to be discussed next).

For experimental rigor and systematic control of any extraneous influences, all participants were treated identically to this point. We were employing a standard experimental technique with a pre-post assessment of the treatment compared to a condition not involving the key personal mastery instructions. The only difference in instructions was in the content of the morning messages that they received. All participants who agreed to be in the study were then assigned either to the Personal Mastery instructions condition or a Health Tips (Comparison Group) condition, providing comparison data against which we could compare our Personal Mastery instructions. Assignment to either of the two conditions was entirely by random selection from a separate code book where names and identification information was removed. In effect, the only significant difference among the participants was the content of the scripted messages they received from the study's automated call system. The participants were informed that their assignment to a condition was entirely at random. The final numbers of participants who completed all steps of the experiment were: 25 into the Personal Mastery condition, and 21 into the Comparison Group condition.

After responding to their initial (pre) questionnaires, the participants were then given an introduction to the steps and procedures to be followed in their particular experimental intervention condition or comparison condition. They were told that it would cover a period of 4 weeks, during which they were to receive an approximately 5-minute telephone call every morning at a time they selected as best for themselves. Our technology involved an automated telephone contact process. We developed carefully scripted messages for each condition of our experimental instructions. These were recorded on tape and then integrated into the telephone contact system. This computerbased automated call system would ring them, wait for their response indicating that they had received the contact, and then the system delivered the scripted message we developed to present the personal mastery or comparison group instructions.

The content of their script contained either the Personal Mastery scripted instructions which we developed from extensive research in the clinical and research literature of personal control and mastery, much of which you now know from having read this book. The Comparison Group's set of health tips was created from extensive review of many public sources of health information: Publicity pamphlets, newspaper comments and reviews, and other sources common in almost all public health publicity campaigns. The information varied over issues about heart health, bone density, weight, nutrition, exercise, weight management, *etc.* These messages carefully avoided making any suggestions about actual personal control thoughts or actions. Thus all participants experienced the technology of the study in exactly the same fashion for the same amount of contact over the same length of time; the key difference was solely the cognitive content of the scripted messages that they received each day: Personal mastery or health information. The fact that the assignment to a condition was random greatly strengthened the power of the experiment to separate out the effects of the technology and the measurement procedures from the therapeutic content of the personal mastery instructions compared to the control participants.

Our experimental design had one additional strength: In addition to the pre-post measurement components of the project, we employed a "daily diary" response procedure conducted online (for the vast majority who had computer access) or with mailed paper assessment questionnaires. Each evening for a month (31 days), the participants were to respond to a number of assessment questions assessing their thoughts and feelings about their reactions to their daily events. They responded each evening, but the telephone instructions began on the third day and ended after 27 days, with the last two days again for reporting feelings for a brief "post" assessment. Again as instructed in the initial meeting, the participants chose a convenient time for them to answer our messages, reporting on their physical and emotional health and feelings during the day. The participants responded online via the internet to these questions or, if they did not have computer access, they were regularly mailed a set of these questionnaires in paper format, with prestamped envelopes to be mailed back to the project staff the following day.

While the pre-post assessment provided information on the overall impact of the experimental treatments, the daily diary responses provided a fine-grained "moving picture" of the participants' on-going thoughts and feelings as they received and processed their daily instructions effects over the 31 days of the project. Both sets of data are significant indicators of any effects our intervention might have (relative to the comparison group's reaction) and I will report here results from both types of assessments.

A final in-person meeting was conducted shortly after the final recorded message. This provided the "post" set of data to compare participants' responses against their initial condition before the experiment commenced to detect any overall change in their condition as a function of the experimental conditions. Also at this meeting the participants were given a stipend, as previously agreed, to compensate them for their time and efforts, a total of $140 for successfully completing all components of the experiment. They also were provided a written description of the logic of the experiment and the rationale for the study: That the daily telephone messages were intended to enhance their control over their lives or, in the case of the control group, how it was expected that the health tips would help them improve their health.

The Personal Mastery Chart of Event Experiences to be Undertaken Daily

In Table 1 below I have presented a model of the instructions table/diagram we presented to the participants as they were receiving their initial instructions. The Table provides some quick and descriptive examples of daily experiences which anyone might experience during their day. Note, of course, that the examples are organized into the 3x2 general categories of events which fit the key dimensions suggested by personal mastery theory and research. This Table was presented to the personal mastery group in our face-to-face first meeting with them. The intent was to give them an overview of their upcoming 27 days of telephone instructions. The participants were encouraged to generate their own personal examples of each of the combinations of control and evaluation, making it more real to them and more relevant to their thoughts and actions during the daily telephone contacts. Since the focus of this chapter is on the personal mastery instructions, I will not add to the reader's burden by discussing the specifics of the Comparison Group condition.

The comparison sample participants did not see this Table and did not know about the Personal Mastery intervention (and *vice versa*). They were presented with a scripted overview of how they would be receiving some health information and tips in the upcoming days of morning telephone calls. The health tips themselves did not follow any pre-set model or structured organization. They were simply brief descriptions of a wide range of things one might think about to keep oneself healthy: good diet, exercise, the necessity of adequate sleep, *etc*.

Measures of Well-Being Assessed in the Experiment

As you will recall from my review of the numerous studies on personal mastery, researchers have employed a wide range of mood and physical and mental health measures that have been shown to be related to personal control. In all of those discussions I glossed over the differences among the dozens numerous measures of physical and mental health. To ease the information overload burden on you the reader I will simply employ here the general terms of "mental health" and "physical health." Since our project involved an entirely new technique

	YOU HAVE CONTROL	SOMEONE OR SOMETHING ELSE IS IN CONTROL
ROUTINE, NEUTRAL THINGS	You started a conversation You drove/biked to work You picked up your newspaper You watered your grass You read a news item	Someone started a conversation A bus or a friend took you to work Someone gave you a newspaper It rained on your grass Someone told you a news item
POSITIVE THINGS YOU CARE ABOUT	For Yourself You bought some ice cream You contacted a good friend You went to a movie For Someone Else You helped someone out You told a funny story You smiled nicely at someone	Someone gave you ice cream A good friend contacted you Someone told you something amazing Someone helped you out Someone told you a funny story Someone smiled nicely at you
NEGATIVE THINGS THAT MATTER TO YOU	For Yourself You did not get your flu shot You drove dangerously You did not check your tires For Someone Else You started an argument You were insensitive to someone You were critical of someone	You got the flu anyway Someone drove dangerously in traffic You had a flat tire Someone started an argument Someone was insensitive to you Someone was critical of you

Table 9.1. Displaying the Daily Experiences Delivered by Telephone to Mastery Project Participants.

of telephone delivery of the mastery manipulation instructions, we did not have definitive predictions about exactly which of these aspects of well-being would show significant effects, so we employed a standard pencil-and-paper instrument for assessing well-being. Certainly we expected that feelings of depression should be an important indicator of our effects. To avoid biasing our results, we explicitly avoided any mention of depression in our initial instructions or the actual scripted daily instructions.

In the research literature, there is a standard assessment scale in near-universal use for studying the physical and emotional components of well-being, the "SF-36" scale.[7] We employed that test and other standard measures of such things as emotions, event activity, and work and social relationships. To present our results most efficiently, I have grouped this discussion into two groups of measures: One set with the global "Pre-Post" to detect overall, more general effects, and the other set of daily diary measures taken at the end of each day for 27 days to detect more specific, day-to-day changes in well-being.

Some Main Results of the Personal Mastery Project

"Pre-Post" Measures: General Perceptions of Physical Health. The SF-36 scale includes a set of 5 items assessing the respondent's thoughts and perceptions of their *general health*. We created a composite (average) score of their responses to questions such as: "In general, would you say your health is "Excellent," "Very Good," "Good," "Fair," or "Poor." Two other questions in this composite were: "I am as healthy as anybody I know," and "I (do not) expect my health to get worse." The results of this analysis are displayed in Figure 9.1. It displays with the solid line the average of the responses of all of the participants in the Personal Mastery group at the beginning and after the conclusion of the daily instructions, and the dashed line shows the averages for all of the participants assigned to the Comparison Group condition for the same two pre-post points of measurement.

As you can see, although the two groups were about equivalent at the time of the Pre measure (the small difference between the two initial scores shown in the figure is not statistically reliable), but by the end of the experiment a month later the Personal

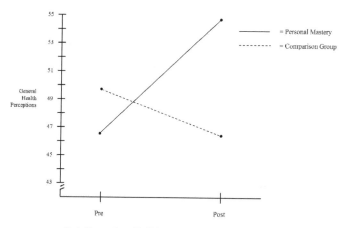

Fig. 1. Change in General Health Perceptions From Before to After the Intervention for Personal Mastery and the Comparison Group Conditions.

Fig. 9.1. Change in General Health Perceptions from Before to After the Intervention for Personal Mastery and the Comparison Group Conditions.

Mastery condition participants were reporting a significant improvement in their perceptions of their own health. The Comparison Group declined somewhat in their perceptions, but the main comparison is between the two groups at the end of the project. The wide separation of the average scores at the conclusion shows that the improvement in the Personal Mastery participants was highly statistically reliable.

"Pre-Post" Measures: Physical Health. We included a large number of measures of the participants' general physical health such as how much bodily pain they had been experiencing in the past month, their energy level, fatigue, and any limitations on their daily activities which had been caused by their physical condition. We found no meaningful differences between the two groups on these measures of physical well-being, so I am not presenting them here. Overall, our data suggest that the Personal Mastery enhancement experience was largely effective in changing perceptions and thoughts toward a more positive tone in the lives of the participants without actually

influencing their ratings of their physical health. Since we did not specifically target their level of physical activity nor did we make any suggestions about medical or bodily well-being, the lack of effect on those measures is easily understandable.

"Pre-Post" Measures: General Perceptions of Mental Health. The SF-36 also contains a subset of items assessing a general level of mental health. The focus here is on a rather broad view of it (as opposed to psychopathology or serious problems in cognitive functioning). The sentence stem asking about mental health asked; "How much time during the past four weeks" followed by such items as "Did you have a lot of energy," "Have you been a very nervous person," "Have you felt downhearted and blue."

The response scale varied from which the respondents were to pick the term most descriptive of how they had been feeling was: "All of the Time," though "Some of the Time" down to "None of the Time."

The results of this scale are presented below in Figure 9.2.

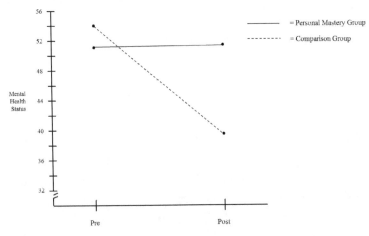

Fig. 2. Change in Mental Health Status From Before to After the Intervention for Personal Mastery and the Comparison Group Conditions.

Fig. 9.2. Change in Mental Health Status From Before to After the Intervention for Personal Mastery and the Comparison Group Conditions.

As you can see there, the Comparison Group declined in their general mental health over the pre-post period of the project, whereas the Personal Mastery group maintained their initial level of mental health with no significant change. It is not clear what might have occurred to the Comparison Group participants during that time. Remember that all participants were randomly assigned to their treatment conditions, and it appears that there was no bias in who got assigned to which group since both groups started out (in the Pre) measure at essentially the same level. The Personal Mastery group appeared to maintain their resilience in their mental health because they did not experience any significant decline in it. In this particular data set, we see the possibility of "no change" being a positive feature of adaptation to life circumstances. A more detailed assessment of the participants' lives during the project over and above what we were able to accomplish in our measurements would have been valuable, and should have developed more thoroughly in any future studies on these variables.

"Pre-Post" Measures: General Perceptions of Mental Functioning. We tested the effects of the intervention treatments with one more generalized measure of the participants' overall mental well-being. We created a composite, generalized score by supplementing the Mental Health scale I just described as a basic measure, and then broadened that measure by adding to it three other different scores from the SF-36. After appropriate statistical explorations to justifying combining the 3 additional scales to the basic mental health scale, we added: (1) a measure of *vitality*. Using the same sentence stem of "How much time during the past 4 weeks... "Did you feel full of pep" and "Did you feel worn out." (2) A second subscale assessed *social functioning*, the extent to which the person's social experiences were compromised by their feelings. The two items assessing this subscale were: "During the past 4 weeks, to what extent have your physical health or emotional problems interfered with

your normal social activities with family, friends, neighbors, or groups" and "...interfered with your social activities (like visiting friends, relatives, *etc*). A third measure, *emotional functioning*, was taken from the SF-36, assessing the extent to which the participants felt that their emotions might have been interfering with their activities. The main item and sub-items for this factor are:

"During the past 4 weeks, have you had any of the following problems with your work or other regular daily activities as a result of any emotional problems (such as feeling depressed or anxious)?

...Cut down on the amount of time you spent on work or other activities.

...Accomplished less than you would like.

...Didn't do work or other activities as carefully as usual."

The results from our analysis of the results of this mental functioning factor are displayed in Figure 9.3.

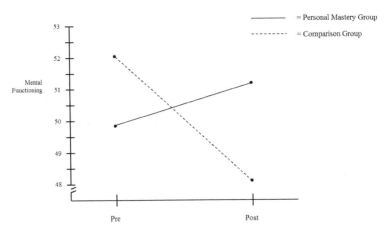

Fig. 3. Change in Mental Functioning From Before to After the Intervention for Personal Mastery and the Comparison Group Conditions.

Fig. 9.3. Change in Mental Functioning From Before to After the Intervention for Personal Mastery and the Comparison Group Conditions.

As you can see, the two groups began the experiment with virtually equivalent levels of general mental functioning. The Comparison Group showed some deterioration in their reports of how they had been functioning mentally, but as we saw in the other two measures, by the end of the project with all of our instructional materials delivered to the participants, the Personal Mastery group reported a higher level of functioning than the Comparison Group. We have no direct evidence to be able to account for the deterioration in the Comparison Group, but it is clear that the Personal Mastery instructions not only prevented any deterioration but actually enhanced their mental functioning.

Participants' Attention and Effort

It was important for us to know the extent to which the participants actually paid attention to the instructions they were receiving each morning and how much they put into actually doing what the instructions were suggesting. After all, we had automatic recordings of the completion of each morning's call, so we knew if they actually picked up the phone to receive their automatic messages (both groups reported receiving nearly 90% of their calls). But of course we had no contact with them during the day and could not assess if they were actually following the suggestions. To get an estimate of that, we asked them a set of brief questions in each of their end-of-day reports:

- *About how much time did you spend today doing what was suggested in your phone call this morning?*
- *About how many times did you think about what was suggested in your phone call this morning?*
- *About how many separate times did you actually do something that was suggested in your phone call this morning?*

Responding on a 4-category response scale moving from low to high amounts of time and attention, the Comparison Group reported significantly less time and effort, while the Personal Mastery group rated at the upper end of the response scale. It seems clear from these results that the Personal Mastery instructions were more engaging and energizing from the participants' point of view. This factor may have played an important role in the overall greater improvement in the mental health measures of those participants.

Did the Project Enhance Personal Mastery Beliefs?

Recall that, before the actual intervention began we asked the participants to respond to the Pearlin and Schooler Personal Mastery Scale which I discussed in Chapter 2 (where I gave you the actual items themselves). Although we did not find changes on every single one of the physical and mental health scales the participants answered, we did find significant effects of the Personal Mastery intervention on some of the more generalized, broader-gauge measures as I have just presented them. Interestingly, however, we found *no* significant difference between the two groups in their sense of personal mastery by the end of the project! The scale is rather stable, as you would want from a trait or personality scale, and that is what we found. In spite of our assumption that it would increase for the Personal Mastery condition, no significant amount of change was found that could be attributed to the intervention. The significant effects that we did find thus changed the participants' emotional and mental health well-being without actually changing their personality structure.

The Daily Diary Assessment

You will recall that in our initial contact with all of the participants in the project, we asked them to respond to a brief screening scale to determine their level of feelings of depression on a standard screening instrument in wide use in psychological research and clinical practice. We screened out from participation many people who were not reporting at least mild-levels of depression, such that all of our participants were reporting some degree of symptoms of depression.

At the end of each day for the full month of the project, the participants responded either online or on mailed paper questionnaires to a set of standard psychological assessment questionnaire items. The focus here was on more momentary, day-to-day assessments of fluctuations in feelings of well-being which might reflect the treatment instructions. This set contained questions tapping into participants' perceptions of their physical health, any injuries or bodily pain, sleep problems, and more cognitive and emotional feelings such as depression, their positive and negative mood at the end of the day, and their thoughts about the stressfulness of their daily experiences. The depression items we employed were: "I felt unable to enjoy life," "I was bothered by feeling down, depressed or hopeless," "I was bothered by little interest or pleasure in doing things." These are direct measures of depressive feelings but with the single exception of the word "hopeless" they do not directly reflect thoughts about personal mastery or control. To show effects on a measure that is not just redundant with the suggestions contained in the intervention wording itself is more convincing evidence of the effectiveness of that intervention.

We took an initial two days' worth of dairy reporting to allow the participants time to get used to the response technique, but that also gave us two measures of their well-being before actually receiving their daily telephone call, a baseline measure. Then the regular pattern of morning call/evening reporting began for the next 27 days. But in the earlier days of the reporting, any effects would not be expected to show up immediately; only a small amount of the intervention suggestions had yet been delivered to the participants in the first two weeks. To conduct our statistical analyses of the data, we clustered days of reporting into units of 3 days each, averaging across those three daily reports into each cluster. This resulted in 11 consecutive data points for each of the two groups. Even condensing into clusters, this graphic is still a lot of data. Since the first set was taken just as the instructions were being delivered, I have arbitrarily plotted for presentation here the results only after half of the instructions, the first half, had been delivered. For convenience of the reader, I decided to plot 15th through 27th intervention days of reports, showing the final effects after the majority and the final days of messages had been received by the participants. We also asked the participants to respond two more days after the final phone call, days 30 and 31, to give us a short view of their reactions after the ending of the morning calls.

To make the effects of the intervention on depression more easily visible, I have developed a figure displaying the results of the assessment of the participants' reports of their feelings of depression across the full range of the 31 days' experience. They are graphed in Figure 4 below. The scores can vary from 1 ("Not at All") to 5 ("Very Much"). This Figure is adapted from our publication report of our original data analyses of this project.[2]

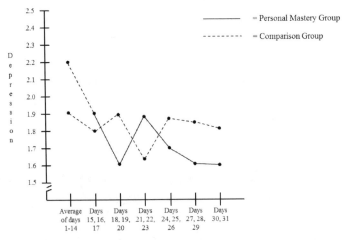

Fig. 4. Changes in Averaged Daily Reports of Depression Across the 31 Days of the Intervention for the Personal Mastery and the Comparison Groups

Fig. 9.4. Changes in Averaged Daily Reports of Depression Across the 31 days of the Intervention for the Personal Mastery and the Comparison Conditions.

I also computed the overall depression ratings for both groups from the very first day of reporting, also creating an average score across the first 14 days of the study, and that average gives you an idea of the degree of depression being reported by the groups when they began the experiment and during the first two weeks of receiving the messages.

Note that the trend to less depression in the Personal Mastery condition is distinct if you consider where they started the project. They were higher in depression than the Comparison Group at the start of the project, but then they declined significantly across the entire course of the telephone messages. The Comparison Group showed much less impressive decline in their reports of their feelings of depression. Recall that assignment of participants to the two conditions of the project was completely at random, so we have to assume a random fluctuation in the Personal Mastery condition at the beginning. But whatever the reason, the final days of the project showed a distinct tendency for the Personal Mastery group to have significantly improved in their depressive feelings than when they started and less than the (randomly assigned) Comparison Group.

Some Summary Thoughts about the Intervention Project

I want to highlight several thoughts about the results and implications of this project. First, it is obvious that not all of the numerous assessment scales we used to test for effects of the intervention showed clear differences between groups. This was particularly noticeable for the many physical health measures we included. Physical conditions such as pain and heart problems are "hard wired" and more difficult to change unless more directive suggestions target them specifically. It was in the more personal realm of emotions, thoughts, and depressive feelings where we were able to detect more impressive effects of the intervention instructions. The Personal Mastery condition was found to have many more positive influences on the participants compared to the Comparison Group condition.

To get an overall picture of these effects, it is important to remember that the actual intervention experienced by the participants in their morning telephone call was quite brief. We took only 5 minutes of our participants' morning time to deliver our instructions in that daily contact. In developing the project we realized that using telephone technology was innovative and had never been tested in the personal mastery/personal control framework, so there was no precedent literature upon which to base our expectations or predictions. We knew of the power of the mastery thinking from all of the thousands of studies on the topic, and we had convincing evidence of the other types of interventions that have been developed as I discussed in Chapter 6. However, we had to keep uppermost in our mind that a morning telephone call with intervention instructions is something completely out of the ordinary for most people's mornings, even if they have freely chosen to participate in it. We wanted to keep the method itself from becoming disruptive or uncomfortable for the participants, so we condensed our daily contacts to the bare minimum of just a few minutes in the morning. It is gratifying to see that we did have a positive influence on the participants' mental health and well-being in some ways, but not in others. Some important dimensions of well-being were positively improved in our Personal Mastery condition even with such a brief treatment. In fact, a number of participants reported informally to us that they looked forward to their morning telephone call, and that they felt that they got a lot out of the experience.

Perhaps one major reason for the success we achieved is that the overall personal mastery treatment is highly *active;* the instructions are highly "behavioral," in the sense of directing the participant to either choose to *do something,* or to actively choose *not to do something,* about any given desirable or undesirable event. While many forms of therapeutic interventions for mental health are highly cognitive or self-focused, the instructions we developed here focused largely on the variable of *choosing* and the variable of *actual action* in the environment of events in which one finds oneself, or creates for oneself. Becoming aware of this distinction no doubt played a role in the outcomes of the study.

At the same time, we cannot claim that any one of the 6 conditions of the 3x2 design had any more effect than any other. The project was a complete, unified set of instructions with no separate assessment of effects coming from any one of the 6 distinct sets of instructions that we implemented. We had no feasible way to conduct any separate assessment of any one of the conditions. To do that more elaborate project would have demanded huge resources and very large samples of participants to provide adequate measurement of those more specific effects. Future research could and should be targeted at trying to find "the active ingredient" in our overall combined set of treatments.

Since the project was time-limited to the one-month period that we set with the participants, the "post" follow-up assessment was only a one-time assessment for determining the longer-term consequences of the project. Also, we had to stop with the daily assessments after the 27th day, so we were not able to continue monitoring the daily effects of the instructions. We do not know if trends for the improvement by the Personal Mastery group participants would continue beyond the post assessment. The trend for that group was encouraging, however. As I said in my Chapter 6 discussion of various personal control intervention studies, there is the suggestion that a "booster shot" of personal mastery and event control suggestions should be encouraged. This could be done at least as a pilot project to see if the improvements which have been found in the various studies can be sustained over the longer-term. The telephone-contact methodology we employed in this project offers an efficient, low-cost way in which those "shots" could be delivered to any number of participants, anywhere, anytime.

What Lessons Have I Learned and
How Have I Been Changed?

I was very impressed by the theory of personal control and mastery when I first read the original articles on it by Julian Rotter, Leonard Pearlin, and the other founders of this field. The approach seemed so realistic and yet so clear in its implications for how we live our daily lives. I quickly adopted its basic ways of thinking early and adapted a personal mastery template for guiding me throughout my life. I hope that this book has induced you to at least be aware of the basic principles of personal mastery and, if you are aware of them, perhaps think about their implications for your own life. The evidence is clear that your well-being can be positively influenced by being in more control of your life and less distressed if you give up trying to control the uncontrollable. Humans are highly adaptable, and switching to accommodation and acceptance is a systematic pathway to achieving your goals even when the world puts up what might otherwise seem uncontrollable.

I find that my adoption of this way of thinking has given me two major principles for how to run my life following a personal mastery approach. I suggest them to you now, at least to think deeply about them and perhaps even try them out. My guess is that they will have a favorable influence in your daily living, as they did mine.

Principle # 1. As I face new or continuing events in my life, although I am aware of events being either desirable or undesirable, I find that my very first thought about either kind of event is, "Can I control it, or is it out of my control?" You may find that thinking about event desirability/undesirability is usually your first reaction to any new event or situation, and those are certainly high in my consciousness as well. But before I begin making any real reactions to an event, or my own mental state of having a desire or a demand (see Chapter 4) my first and most important thought is, "What can I do about this?" One's actions are very different depending on the answer to that question. The Reinhold Niebuhr Serenity Prayer that I presented in my Preface has turned out to be profound indeed. As we near the end of this book it should be clear why I think science has fully supported his basic insights and has extended it into many novel and fruitful new pathways for us all.

Principle # 2. Once I know the answer to the first question, I am now able to organize my reactions in the framework of "primary control" of changing my world and alternative paths for control in the form of adapting myself to "things" outside of my personal control originally proposed by Weisz, and Samuel Snyder (see Chapter 3). Controllability is often difficult and achieving our goals sometimes is so difficult that we want to retreat, give up, to change our mind about the event. But "retreating" need not be the end of the question, and giving up your goals may be easy, but that potentially undermines your sense of personal control. You always have ways of coping, of choosing alternative paths and/or alternative responses that can still keep you on track for achieving your goals. The old adage "If at first you don't succeed, try, try again" is useful but probably needs to be rephrased to "If at first you don't succeed, drop the original "try" and move to an alternative... your resilience and adaptability gives you a huge range of coping devices... so be creative, not stuck in an unrewarding futility." "You need not give up your goals, just give up poor mechanisms to achieve them." I know it does not sound nearly as musical, but it is realistic and it works. Pragmatism based on tested and valid scientific principles strikes me as much more encouraging for creating and maintaining our well-being based on the best scientific evidence that we now have. You now have the power to make the Serenity Prayer a real part of who you are and how you can best live your life to the fullest.

References

Introduction References

1. Fredrickson, B. (2001). The role of positive emotions in positive psychology: The broaden-and-build theory of positive emotions. *American Psychologist, 56*, 218-226.
2. Reich, J. W., Zautra, A. J., & Hall, J. S. (Eds.). (2010). *Handbook of Adult Resilience: Concepts, Methods, and Applications*. New York: Guilford Publications.
3. Zautra, A. J., Davis, M. E., Reich, J. W., Sturgeon, J. A., Arewasikporn, A., & Tennen, H. (2012). Phone-based interventions with automated mindfulness and mastery messages improve the daily functioning for depressed middle-aged community residents. *Journal of Psychotherapy Integration, 22*, 206-228.
4. Lyubomirsky, S. (2013). *The myths of happiness: What should make you happy but doesn't. What shouldn't make you happy, but does*. New York: Press Penguin.
5. Gilbert, D. (2007). *Stumbling on happiness*. New York: Vintage Books.
6. Reich, J. W., Zautra, A., J., & Davis, M. C. (2003). Dimensions of affect relationships: Models and their integrative implications. *Review of General Psychology, 7*, 66-83.
7. White, R. (1959). Motivation reconsidered: The concept of competence. *Psychological Review, 66*, 297-333.

Chapter 1 References

1. Maslow, A. (1987). *Motivation and personality*. New York: Harper and Row.

Chapter 2 References

1. Skinner, E. (1996). A guide to constructs of control. *Journal of Personality and Social Psychology, 71*, 549-570.

2. Bandura, A. (1977). Self-efficacy: Toward a unified theory of behavior. *Psychological Review, 84,* 191-215.

3. Bandura, A. (1989). Human agency in social cognitive theory. *American Psychologist, 44,* 1175-1184.

4. Weisz, J., & Stipek, D. J. (1982). Competence, contingency, and the development of perceived control. *Human Development, 25,* 250-281.

5. Abramson, L., Y, Seligman, M.E. P., & Teasdale, J. D. (1978). Learned helplessness in humans. *Journal of Abnormal Psychology, 87,* 49-74.

6. Skinner, E. A. (1995). *Perceived control, motivation, and coping.* Thousand Oaks, CA: Sage.

7. Rotter, J. B. (1966). Generalized expectancies for internal versus external locus of control. *Psychological Monographs, 80, 1, (Whole No. 609).*

8. Pearlin, L. I., & Schooler, C. (1978). The structure of coping. *Journal of Health and Social Behavior, 19,* 2-21.

9. Wallston, B. S., Wallston, K. A., Kaplan, G. D., & Maides, S. A. (1976). Development and validation of the health locus of control (HLC) scale. *Journal of Consulting and Clinical Psychology, 44,* 580-585.

10. Keyson, M. & Janda, L. (1972). *Untitled health locus of drinking control scale.* Unpublished manuscript, St. Luke's Hospital, Phoenix, AZ. Reported in Donovan, D., & O'Leary, M. (1978). The drinking-related locus of control scale. *Journal of Studies on Alcohol, 39,* 759-784.

11. Strickland, B. R. (1989) Internal-external control expectancies. *American Psychologist, 44,* 1-12.

12. Strickland, B. R. (1978). Internal-external expectances and health-related behaviors. *Journal of Consulting and Clinical Psychology, 46,* 1192-1211.

13. Lachman, M. E., Neupert, S. D., & Agrigoroaei, S. (2011). The relevance of control beliefs for health and aging. Chapter 11 in K. W. Schaie, & S. L. Willis (Eds.) *Handbook*

of the Psychology of Aging, 7th ed. (pp. 175-190). New York: Elsevier.

14. Wallston, B. S., & Wallston, K.A. (1978). Locus of control and health: A review of the literature. *Health Education Monographs, 6*, 107-117.
15. Hoge, E. A., Austin, E. D., & Pollack, M. H (2006). Resilience: Research evidence and conceptual considerations for posttraumatic stress disorder. *Depression and Anxiety, 24*, 134-152.
16. Ozer, E.M., & Bandura, A. (1990). Mechanisms governing empowerment effects. A self-efficacy analysis. *Journal of Personality and Social Psychology, 58*, 472-486.
17. Lachman, M. E., & Firth, K. M. (2004). The adaptive value of feeling in control during midlife. In O. G. Brim, C. D. Ryff, & R. Kessler (Eds). *How healthy are we? A national study of well-being at midlife.* (pp. 320-349). Chicago: University of Chicago Press.
18. Strickland, B. R. (1979). Internal-external expectancies and cardiovascular functioning. In L. C. Perlmuter & R. A. Monty (Eds.), *Choice and perceived control.* Hillsdale, NJ: Erlbaum.
19. Rodin, J., & Timko, C. (1992). Sense of control, aging, and health. In M. G. Ory, R. P. Abeles, & P. D. Lipman, (Eds.), *Aging, health, and behavior.* Newbury Park, NJ: Sage.
20. Butts, S. V., & Chotlos, J. (1973). A comparison of alcoholics and nonalcoholics on perceived locus of control. *Quarterly Journal of Studies on Alcohol, 34*, 1327-1332.
21. Donovan, D. M., & O'Leary, M. R. (1978). The drinking-related locus of control scale: Reliability, factor structure, and validity. *Journal of Studies on Alcohol, 39*, 759-784.
22. Benassi, V. A., Sweeney, P.D., & C. L. Dufour (1988). Is there a relation between locus of control orientation and depression? *Journal of Abnormal Psychology, 97*, 357-367.
23. Cheng, C., Cheung,S-f., Chio, J.H-m., & Chan, Man-p. (2013). Cultural meaning of perceived control: A meta-analysis

of locus of control and psychological symptoms across 18 cultural regions. *Psychological Bulletin, 139*, 152-188.

24. Sandler, I. N., & Lakey, B. (1982). Locus of control as a stress moderator: The role of control perceptions and social support. *American Journal of Community Psychology, 10*, 65-80.

25. Pudrovska, T., Schieman, S., Pearlin, L. I., and Nguyen, K. (2005). The sense of mastery as a mediator and moderator in the association between economic hardship and health in late life. *Journal of Aging and Health, 17*, 634-660.

26. Price, R. H., Choi, J. N., & Vinokur, A. D. (2002). Links in the chain of adversity following job loss: How financial strain and loss of personal control lead to depression, impaired functioning, and poor health. *Journal of Occupational Health Psychology, 7*, 302-312.

27. Roepke, S. K., Mausbach, B.R., van Kanel, R., Ancoli-Israel, S., Harmell, A. L., Dimsdale, J. E., Aschbacher, K.,Mills, P. J., Patterson, T. L., & Grant, I. (2009).The moderating role of personal mastery on the relationship between caregiving status and multiple dimensions of fatigue. *International Journal of Geriatric Psychiatry, 24*, 1453-1462.

28. Infurna, F. J., Gerstorf, D., Ram, N., Schupp, J., & Wagner, G. G. (2011). Long-term antecedents and outcomes of perceived control. *Psychology and Aging, 26*, 559-575.

29. Penninx, B. W., J. H, van Tilburg, T., Boeke, J. P., Deeg, D. J.K., Kriegsman, D. M W, & van Eijk, J. T. M. (1998). Effects of social support and personal coping resources on depressive symptoms: Different for various chronic diseases? *Health Psychology, 17*, 551-558.

30. Ryckman, R. M. (1979). Perceived locus of control and task performance. In L. C. Perlmuter & R. A. Monty (Eds.), *Choice and perceived control*. Hillsdale, NJ: Erlbaum.

31. Schneider, J. M. (1968). Skill versus chance activity preference and locus of control. *Journal of Consulting and Clinical Psychology, 32*, 333-337.

32. Ducette, J., & Wolk, S. (1972). Locus of control and extreme behavior. *Journal of Consulting and Clinical Psychology, 39*, 253-258.

33. Crowne, D. P., & Liverant, S. (1963). Conformity under varying conditions of personal commitment. *Journal of Abnormal and Social Psychology, 66*, 547-555.

34. Hoff, E-H., & Hohner, H-U. (1986). Occupational careers, work, and control. In M. M. Baltes & P. B. Baltes (Eds.), *The psychology of control and aging*. Hillsdale, NJ. Erlbaum.

35. Broedling, L. A. (1975). Relationship of internal-external control to work motivation and performance in an expectancy model. *Journal of Applied Psychology, 60*, 65-70.

36. Kilman, P. R., Albert, B.M., & Sotile, W.M. (1975). Relationship between locus of control, structure of therapy, and outcomes. *Journal of Consulting and Clinical Psychology, 43*, 588.

37. Brownell, P. (1982). The effects of personality-situation congruence in a managerial context: Locus of control and budgetary participation. *Journal of Personality and Social Psychology, 42*, 753-763.

38. Bryant, F. (1989). A four-factor model of perceived control: Avoiding, coping, obtaining, and savoring. *Journal of Personality, 57*, 773-797.

39. Grossman, R. M. (1986). *Attributions of Responsibility and Social Support*. Unpublished doctoral dissertation, Arizona State University, Tempe.

40. Reich, J. W., & Zautra, A. J. (1995). Spouse encouragement of self-reliance and other-reliance in rheumatoid arthritis patients. *Journal of Behavioral Medicine, 18*, 249-260.

41. Reich, J. W., & Zautra, A. J. (1995). Other-reliance encouragement effects in female rheumatoid arthritis patients. *Journal of Social and Clinical Psychology, 14*, 119-133.

42. Helgeson, V. S. (1993). The onset of chronic illness: Its effect on the patient-spouse relationship. *Journal of Social and Clinical Psychology, 12*, 406-428.

43. Shapiro, D. H., Schwartz, C.E., & Astin, J. A. (1996). Controlling ourselves, controlling our world: Psychology's role in understanding positive and negative consequences of seeking and gaining control. *American Psychologist, 51*, 1213-1230.
44. Rothbaum, F., Weisz, J. R., and Snyder, S. S. (1984). Changing the world and changing the self: A two-process model of perceived control. *Journal of Personality and Social Psychology, 39*, 5-37.
45. Morling, B., & Evered, S. (2007). The construct formerly known as secondary control: Reply to Skinner (2007). *Psychological Bulletin, 133*, 917-919.
46. Skinner, E. (2007). Secondary control critiques: Is it Secondary: Is it control? Comment on Morling and Evered (2006). *Psychological Bulletin, 133*, 911-916.
47. Hodges, D. (2014). Music as an agent of resilience. In M. Kent, M. C. Davis, and J. W. Reich (Eds,), *The resilience handbook: Approaches to stress and trauma.* New York: Routledge.
48. Brandstetter, J., & Rothermund, K. (2002). The life course dynamics of goal pursuit and good adjustment: A two-process framework. *Developmental Research, 22*, 117-150.
49. Rodin, J. (1986). Health, control, and aging. In M. M. Baltes & P. B. Baltes (Eds.), *The psychology of control and aging.* Hillsdale, NJ: Erlbaum.
50. Wong, P. T., & Sproule, C. F. (1988). An attributional analysis of the locus of control construct and the Trent Attribution Profile. In H. Lefcourt (Ed.), *Research with the locus of control construct. Vol. 3. Extensions and limitations.* NewYork: Academic Press.

Chapter 3 References

1. Holmes, T. H., & Rahe, R. H. (1967). The social readjustment rating scale. *Journal of Psychosomatic Research, 11*, 213-218.
2. Markush, R. E, & Favero, R. V. (1974). Epidemiological assessment of stressful life events, depressed mood, and

psychophysiological symptoms: A preliminary report. In Dohrenwend, B. S., & Dohrenwend, B.P. (Eds.), *Stressful life events: Their nature and effects*. New York: Wiley.

3. Myers, J. K., Lindenthal, J. J., & Pepper, M. P. (1974). Social class, life events, and psychiatric symptoms. A longitudinal study. In Dohrenwend, B. S., & Dohrenwend (Eds.), *Stressful life events: Their nature and effects*. New York:

4. Rahe, R.H., & Lind, E. (1971). Psychosocial factors and sudden cardiac arrest: A pilot study. *Journal of Psychosomatic Research, 15*, 19-24.

5. Dorian, B., & Garfinkle, P. E. (1987). Stress, immunity, and illness – A review. *Psychological Medicine, 17*, 387-392.

6. Perretti, P. O., & Wilson, C. (1975). Voluntary and involuntary retirement of aged males and their effect on emotional satisfaction, usefulness, self-image, emotional stability, and interpersonal relationships. *The International Journal of Aging and Human Development, 6*, 131-138.

7. Smith, R. T., & Brand, F. N. (1975). Effects of enforced relocation on life adjustment in a nursing home. *The International Journal of Aging and Human Development, 6*, 249-259.

8. Bay, R.C., & Braver, S. L. (1990). Perceived control of the divorce settlement process and interparental conflict. *Family Relations, 39*, 382-387.

9. Braver, S. L., Wolchik, S.A, Sandler, I. N., Sheets, V. L., Fogas, B., & Bay, R. C. (1993). A longitudinal study of noncustodial parents: Parents without children. *Journal of Family Psychology, 7*, 9-23.

10. Kanner, A. D., Coyne, J. C., Schaefer, C. & Lazarus, R. S. (1981). Comparison of two modes of stress measurement: Daily hassles and uplifts versus major life events. *Journal of Behavioral Medicine, 4*, 1-39.

11. Zautra, A. J., Guarnaccia, C. A., & Dohrenwewnd, B.P. (1986). Measuring small life events. *American Journal of Community Psychology, 14*, 629-655.

12. Zautra, A. J., Guarnaccia, C. A., Reich, J. W., & Dohrenwend, B. P. (1988). The contributions of small events to stress and distress. In L. Cohen (Ed.), *Life events and psychological functioning: Theoretical and methodological issues*. Newbury Park, CA. Sage.

13. Pillow, D. R., Zautra, A. J., & Sandler, I. (1996). Major life events and minor stressors: Identifying mediational links in the stress process. *Journal of Personality and Social Psychology, 79*, 381-394.

14. Zautra, A. J., & Reich, J. W. (1983). Life events and perceptions of life quality: Developments in a two-factor approach. *Journal of Community Psychology, 11*, 121-132.

15. Reich, J. W., Zautra, A. J., & Davis, M. C. (2003). Dimensions of affect relationships: Models and their integrative implications. *Review of General Psychology, 7*, 66-83.

16. Potter, P. T., Zautra A. J., & Reich, J. W. (2000). Stressful events and information processing dispositions moderate the relationship between positive and negative affect: Implications for pain patients. *Annals of Behavioral Medicine, 22*, 191-198.

17. Zautra, A. J. (2003). *Emotions, stress, and health*. New York: Oxford.

18. Cacioppo, J. T., & Berntson, G. G. (1994). Relationship between attitudes and evaluative space: A critical review, with emphasis on the separability of positive and negative substrates. *Psychological Bulletin, 115*, 401-423.

19. Herzberg, F. (1966). *Work and the nature of man*. Cleveland: World Publishing.

20. DeCharms, R. (1976). *Enhancing motivation in the classroom*. New York: Irvington, Halstead-Wiley

21. Zautra, A.J., & Reich. J. W. (1980). Positive life events and reports of well-being: Some useful distinctions. *American Journal of Community Psychology, 8*, 657-669.

22. Strand, E. B., Reich, J. W., & Zautra, A.J. (2007). Control and causation as factors in the affective value of positive events. *Cognitive Therapy and Research, 31*, 503-519.

23. Reich, J. W., & Zautra, A. J. (1983). Demands and desires in daily life: Some influences on well-being. *American Journal of Community Psychology, 11*, 41-58.

24. Reich, J. W., McCall, M., Grossman, R., Zautra, A. J., & Guarnaccia, C.A. (1988). Demands, desires, and well-being: An assessment of events, responses, and outcomes. *Journal of Community Psychology, 16*, 392-402.

25. James, W. (1890). *The principles of psychology.* Chapter 4 "Habits." New York: Henry Holt.

26. Thompson, S. C. (1981). Will it hurt less if I can control it? A complex answer to a simple question. *Psychological Bulletin, 90*, 89-101.

27. Zautra, A. J., Guarnaccia, C. A., & Reich, J. W. (1989). The effects of daily life events on negative affective states. In P. C. Kendall & D. Watson (Eds.) *Anxiety and depression: Overlapping features.* New York: Academic Press.

28. Luhmann, M., & Eid, M. (2009). Does it really feel the same? Changes in life Satisfaction following repeated life events. *Journal of Personality and Social Psychology, 97*, 363-381.

29. Wright, M., Zautra, A. J., & Braver, S. L. (1985). Distortion in control attributions for real life events. *Journal of Research in Personality, 19*, 54-71.

30. Rothbaum, F., Weisz, J. R., and Snyder, S. S. (1982). Changing the world and changing the self: A two-process model of perceived control. *Journal of Personality and Social Psychology, 42*, 5-37.

Chapter 4 References

1. Mirowsky, J., & Ross, C. E. (1990). Control or defense: Depression and the sense of control over good and bad outcomes. *Journal of Health and Social Behavior, 31*, 71-86.

2. Bulman, R. J., & Wortman, C.B. (1977). Atribution of blame and coping in the "real world": Severe accident victims react

to their lot. *Journal of Personality and Social Psychology, 35,* 351-363.

3. Affleck, G., Tennen, H., Pfeiffer,C., & Fifield, J. (1987). Appraisals of control and predictability in adapting to a chronic disease. *Journal of Personality and Social Psychology, 53,* 273-279.

4. Nicassio, P. M., Wallston, K. A., Callahan, L. F., Herbert, M, & Pincus, T. (1985). The measurement of helplessness in rheumatoid arthritis: The development of the Arthritis Helplessness Index. *Journal of Rheumatology, 12,* 462-467.

5. Taylor, S. E., Helgeson, V .S, Reed, G. M., & Skokan, L. A. (1991). Self-generated feelings of control and adjustment to physical illness. *Journal of Social Issues, 47,* 91-109.

6. Janoff-Bulman, R. (1979). Characterological versus behavioral self-blame: Inquiries into depression and rape. *Journal of Personality and Social Psychology, 37,* 1798-1809.

7. Frazier, P. A. (1990). Victim attributions and post-rape trauma. *Journal of Personality and Social Psychology, 90,* 298-304.

8. Felton, B., & Kahana, E. (1974). Adjustment and situationally-bound locus of control among institutionalized aged. *Journal of Gerontology, 29,* 295-301.

9. Baltes, M. M., & Reisenzein, R. (1986). The social world in long-term care institutions: Psychosocial control toward dependency. In M. M. Baltes & P. B. Baltes (Eds.), *The psychology of control and aging.* Chapter 12. Hillsdale, NJ: Erlbaum.

10. Wolk, S. (1976). Situational constraint as a moderator of the locus of control-adjustment relationship. *Journal of Consulting and Clinical Psychology, 44,* 420-427.

11. Abramowitz, C. V., Abramowitz, S. L., Roback, H. B., & Jackson, C. (1974). Differential effectiveness of directive and nondirective group therapies as a function of client internal-

external control. *Journal of Consulting and Clinical Psychology,* *42,* 849-853.

12. Seligman, M. E. P., & Maier, S. F. (1967). Failure to escape traumatic shock. *Journal of Experimental Psychology, 74,* 1-9.

13. Hiroto, D. (1974). Locus of control and learned helplessness. *Journal of Experimental Psychology, 102,* 187-193.

14. Glass, D. C., & Singer, J. E. (1972). *Urban stress.* New York: Academic Press.

15. Glass, D. C., Singer, J. E., & Friedman, L. N. (1969). Psychic cost of adaptation to an environmental stressor. *Journal of Personality and Social Psychology, 12,* 200-210.

Chapter 5 References

1. Reich, J. W., & Zautra, A. J. (1988). Direct and stress-moderating effects of positive life experiences. In L. Cohen (Ed.), *Life events and psychological functioning: Theoretical and methodological issues.* Newbury Park, CA: Sage.

2. Brickman, P., & Campbell, D. T. (1971). Hedonic relativism and planning the good society. In M. H. Appley (Ed.), *Adaptation-level theory: A symposium.* New York: Academic Press.

3. Helson, H. (1964). *Adaptation-level theory.* New York: Harper and Row.

4. Zautra, A. J., & Reich, J. W. (1980). Positive life events and reports of well-being: Some useful distinctions. *American Journal of Community Psychology, 8,* 657-670.

5. deCharms, R. (1976). *Enhancing motivation in the classroom.* New York: Irvington-Halsted, Wiley.

6. Iyengar, S. (2010). *The art of choosing.* New York: Hachette Book Group.

7. Lepper, M. R., Green, D., & Nisbett, R. E. (1973). Undermining children's intrinsic interest with extrinsic reward: A test of the "overjustification" hypothesis. *Journal of Personality and Social Psychology, 28,* 129-137.

8. www.abcbodybuilding.com" or www.drclue.com/free-resources/can-people-really-be-motivated/

9. Reich, J. W., & Gutierres, S. E. (1987). Life event and treatment attributions in drug abuse and rehabilitation. *The American Journal of Drug and Alcohol Abuse, 13,* 69-90.

10. Brown, S. L., Smith, D. M., Schulz, R., Kabeto, M., Ubel, P., Yee, J...Langa, K. (2009). Caregiving and decreased mortality in a national sample of older adults *Psychological Science, 20,* 488-494.

11. Brown, S. L., Nesse, R., Vinokur, A. D., & Smith, D.M. (2003). Providing social support may be more beneficial than receiving it: Results from a prospective study of mortality. *Psychological Science, 14,* 320-327.

12. Okun, M. A., August, K. J, Rook, K.S., & Newsom, J. T. (2010). Does volunteering moderate the relation between functional imitations and mortality? *Social Science and Medicine, 71,* 1662-1668.

13. Midlarsky, E., & Kahana, E. (1994). *Altruism in later life.* Thousand Oaks, CA. Sage.

14. Langer, E. (1975). The illusion of control. *Journal of Personality and Social Psychology, 32,* 311-328.

15. Kahneman, D. (2011). *Thinking, fast and slow.* New York: Farrar, Straus, and Giroux.

16. Brickman, P., Coates, D., & Janoff-Bulman, R. (1978). Lottery winners and accident victims: Is happiness relative? *Journal of Personality and Social Psychology, 36,* 917-927.

17. Diener, E., Lucas, R. E., & Scollon, C.N. (2006). Beyond the hedonic treadmill: Revising the adaptation theory of well-being. *American Psychologist, 61,* 305-314

18. Winkelmann, R., Oswald, A.J., & Powdthavee, N. (2010). *What happens to people after winning the lottery?* Manuscript submitted for publication.

19. Gardner, J., & Oswald, A. J. (2007). Money and mental well-being: A longitudinal study of medium-sized lottery wins. *Journal of Health Economics, 26,* 49-60.

20. Apouey, B. J., & Clark, A. (2008). *Winning big but feeling no better? The effect of lottery prizes on physical and mental health.* Manuscript submitted for publication.

21. Arkes, H. A., Joyner, C.A., Pezzo, M. V., & Gradwhol, J. (1994). The psychology of windfall gains. *Organizational Behavior and Human Decision Processes, 59,* 331-347.

22. Kahneman, D., Krueger, A. B., Schkade, D., Schwarz, N., & Stone, A. A. (2006). Would you be happier if you were richer? A focusing illusion. *Science, 30 June, 2006, 312,* 1908-1910.

23. Glass, D. C., Singer, J. E., & Friedman, L. N. (1969). Psychic cost of adaptation to an environmental stressor. *Journal of Personality and Social Psychology, 12,* 200-210.

24. Perlmuter, L. C., & Langer, E. J. (1982). The effects of behavioral monitoring on the perception of control. *Clinical Gerontology, 1,* 37-43.

25. Emerson, R. W. (1840). *Essays: First Series. "Compensation."* New York: Hurst. (p. 40). 200-210.

Chapter 6 References

1. Jacobson, N. S., Dobson, K. S., Truax, M., Addis, M. E., Koerner, K., Prince, S. E. (1996). A component analysis of cognitive-behavioral treatment for depression. *Journal of Consulting and Clinical Psychology, 64,* 295-304.

2. DeCharms, R. (1968). *Personal causation.* New York: Academic Press.

3. DeCharms, R. (1972). Personal causation in the schools. *Journal of Applied Social Psychology, 2,* 95-113.

4. Reich, J. W., & Zautra, A. J. (1981). Life events and personal causation: Some relationships with satisfaction and distress. *Journal of Personality and Social Psychology, 41,* 1002-1012.

5. Reich, J. W., & Zautra, A. J. (1989). A perceived control intervention for at-risk older adults. *Psychology and Aging, 4,* 415-424.

6. Reich, J., & Zautra, A. J (1990). Dispositional control beliefs and the consequences of a control-enhancing intervention. *Journal of Gerontology: Psychological Sciences, 45,* P46-P51.

7. Langer, E. J., & Rodin, J. (1976). The effects of choice and enhanced personal responsibility for the aged: A field experiment in an institutional setting. *Journal of Personality and Social Psychology, 34,* 191-198.

8. Rodin, J., & Langer, E. J. (1977). Long-term effects of a control-relevant intervention with the institutionalized aged. *Journal of Personality and Social Psychology, 35,* 897-902.

9. Slivinske, L. R., & Fitch, V. L. (1987). The effect of control enhancing intervention on the well-being of elderly individuals living in retirement communities. *The Gerontologist, 27,* 176-180.

10. Mercer, S., & Kane, R. A. (1979). Helplessness and hopelessness among the institutionalized aged: An experiment. *Health and Social Work, 4,* 90-116.

11. Banziger, G., & Roush, S. (1983). Nursing home for the birds: A control-relevant intervention with bird feeders. *The Gerontologist, 23,* 527-531.

12. Schulz, R. (1976). Effects of control and predictability on the physical and psychological well-being of the institutionalized aged. *Journal of Personality and Social Psychology, 33,* 563-573.

13. Schulz, R., & Hanusa, B. (1978). Long-term effects of control and predictability-enhancing interventions: Findings and ethical issues. *Journal of Personality and Social Psychology, 36,* 1194-1201.

14. Haemmerlie, F. M., & Montgomery, R. L. (1987). Self-perception theory, salience of behavior, and a control-enhancing program for the elderly. *Journal of Social and Clinical Psychology, 5,* 313-329.

Chapter 7 References

1. Zautra, A.J., & Reich. J. W. (1980). Positive life events and reports of well-being: Some useful distinctions. *American Journal of Community Psychology, 8*, 657-669.
2. Strand, E. B., Reich, J. W., & Zautra, A.J. (2007). Control and causation as factors in the affective value of positive events. *Cognitive Therapy and Research, 31*, 503-519.
3. Gardner, H. (1961). *A thousand clowns*. New York: Random House.
4. Glass, D. C., Singer, J. E., & Friedman, L. N. (1969). Psychic cost of adaptation to an environmental stressor. *Journal of Personality and Social Psychology, 12*, 200-210.
5. Perlmuter, L. C., & Langer, E. J. (1982). The effects of behavioral monitoring on the perception of control. *Clinical Gerontology, 1*, 37-43.
6. Brickman, P., & Campbell, D. T. (1971). Hedonic relativism and planning the good society. In M. H. Appley (Ed.), *Adaptation-level theory: A symposium*. New York: Academic Press.
7. Zautra, A. J., & Reich, J. W. (1980). Positive life events and reports of well-being: Some useful distinctions. *American Journal of Community Psychology, 8*, 657-670.
8. Brickman, P., Coates, D., & Janoff-Bulman, R. (1978). Lottery winners and accident victims: Is happiness relative? *Journal of Personality and Social Psychology, 36*, 917-927.
9. Iyengar, S. (2010). *The art of choosing*. New York: Hachette Book Group.
10. Lepper, M. R., Green, D., & Nisbett, R. E. (1973). Undermining children's intrinsic interest with extrinsic reward: A test of the "overjustification" hypothesis. *Journal of Personality and Social Psychology, 28*, 129-137.
11. Mirowsky, J., & Ross, C. E. (1990). Control or defense: Depression and the sense of control over good and bad outcomes. *Journal of Health and Social Behavior, 31*, 71-86.

12. Bulman, R. J., & Wortman, C.B. (1977). Attribution of blame and coping in the "real world": Severe accident victims react to their lot. *Journal of Personality and Social Psychology, 35,* 351-363.

13. Frazier, P. A. (1990). Victim attributions and post-rape trauma. *Journal of Personality and Social Psychology, 90,* 298-304.

14. Affleck, G., Tennen, H., Pfeiffer,C., & Fifield, J. (1987). Appraisals of control and predictability in adapting to a chronic disease. *Journal of Personality and Social Psychology, 53,* 273-279.

15. Reich, J. W., & Gutierres, S. E. (1987). Life event and treatment attributions in drug abuse and rehabilitation. *The American Journal of Drug and Alcohol Abuse, 13,* 69-90.

16. Brown, S. L., Smith, D. M., Schulz, R., Kabeto, M., Ubel, P., Yee, J., Langa, K. (2009). Caregiving and decreased mortality in a national sample of older adults. *Psychological Science, 20,* 488-494

17. Brown, S. L., Nesse, R., Vinokur, A. D., & Smith, D. M. (2003). Providing social support may be more beneficial than receiving it: Results from a prospective study of mortality. *Psychological Science, 14,* 320-327.

18. Okun, M. A., August, K., J, Rook, K. S., & Newsom, J. T. (2010). Does volunteering moderate the relation between functional imitations and mortality? *Social Science and Medicine, 71,* 1662-1668.

19. Miller, G. A. (1969). Psychology as a means of promoting human welfare. *American Psychologist, 24,* 1063-1075.

Chapter 8 References

1. James, W. (1890). *The principles of psychology.* Chapter 4. "Habits." New York: Henry Holt.

2. Masten, A. (2001). Ordinary magic: Resilience processes in development. *American Psychologist, 56,* 227-238.

3. Reich, J. W. (2006). Three psychological principles of resilience in natural disasters. *Disaster Prevention and Management, 15,* 793-798.
4. Rothbaum, F., Weisz, J. R., and Snyder, S. S. (1984). Changing the world and and changing the self: A two-process model of perceived control. *Journal of Personality and Social Psychology, 39,* 5-37.
5. Baron, R., & Ransberger, V. (1978). Ambient temperature and the occurrence of collective violence: The "long, hot summer" revisited. *Journal of Personality and Social Psychology, 36,* 351-360.
6. Anderson, C., A., Bushman, B. J., & Groom, R. W. (1997). Hot years and serious and deadly assault: Empirical test of the heat hypothesis. *Journal of Personality and Social Psychology, 73,* 1213-1223.
7. Myers, D. (2007). *Psychology.* New York: Worth.
8. Brehm, J. (1966). *A theory of psychological reactance.* New York: Academic Press.
9. Worchel, S., & Brehm, J. (1970). Effects of threats to attitudinal freedom as a function of agreement with the communicator. *Journal of Personality and Social Psychology, 14,* 18-22.
10. Reich, J. W., & Robertson, J. (1979). Reactance and norm appeal in anti-littering messages. *Journal of Applied Social Psychology, 9,* 91-101.
11. Hepworth, J. T., & West, S. G. (1988). Lynchings and the economy: A time-series reanalysis of Hovland and Sears (1940). *Journal of Personality and Social Psychology, 55,* 239-247.
12. Reich, J. W., & Zautra, A. J. (1995). Spouse encouragement of self-reliance and other-reliance in rheumatoid arthritis patients. *Journal of Behavioral Medicine, 18,* 249-260.
13. Reich, J. W., & Zautra, A. J. (1995). Other-reliance encouragement effects in female rheumatoid arthritis patients. *Journal of Social and Clinical Psychology, 14,* 119-133.

14. Cialdini, R. B. (2004). *Influence: Science and practice*. (4th Ed.). Boston: Allyn and Bacon.
15. Trickett, P. K., & McBride-Chang. (1995). The developmental impact of different forms of child abuse and neglect. *Developmental Review, 15*, 311-337.
16. Langlois, J., H., Ritter, J. M., Casey, R. J., and Sawin, D. B. (1995). Infant attractiveness predicts maternal behaviors and attitudes. *Developmental Psychology, 31*, 464-472.
17. Dion, K. K., Berscheid, E., & Walster, E. (1982). What is beautiful is good. *Journal of Personality and Social Psychology, 24*, 285-290.
18. Eagly, A. J., Ashmore, R. D., Makhijani, M. G., & Longo, L. C. (1991). What is beautiful is good, but...: A meta-analytic review of research on the physical attractiveness stereotype. *Psychological Bulletin, 110*, 109-128.
19. Goffman, E., (1963). *Stigma: Notes on the management of spoiled identity*. Englewood Cliffs, NJ: Prentice-Hall.

Chapter 9 References

1. Reich, J. W., McCall, M., Grossman, R., Zautra, A. J., & Guarnaccia, C.A. (1988). Demands, desires, and well-being: An assessment of events, responses, and outcomes. *Journal of Community Psychology, 16*, 392-402.
2. Reich, J. W., & Zautra, A. J. (1981). Life events and personal causation: Some relationships with satisfaction and distress. *Journal of Personality and Social Psychology, 41*, 1002-1012.
3. This project was supported by NIA Grant RO1-AG-6026006 NIA Supplement Grant RO1-AG-0266006. The author gratefully acknowledges the support of the Arizona State University Office of Research and Sponsored Projects, Dr. Rick Shangraw, Vice-President.
4. Zautra, A. J., Davis, M.C. Reich, J. W., Sturgeon, J. A., & Arewasikporn (2012). Phone-based interventions with

   automated mindfulness and mastery messages improve the daily functioning for depressed middle-aged community residents. *Journal of Psychotherapy Integration, 22,* 206-228.

5. Benassi, V. A., Sweeney, P.D., & C. L. Dufour (1988). Is there a relation between locus of control orientation and depression? *Journal of Abnormal Psychology, 97,* 357-367.

6. Cheng, C., Cheung,S-f., Chio, J.H-m., & Chan, Man-p. (2013). Cultural meaning of perceived control: A meta-analysis of locus of control and psychological symptoms across 18 cultural regions. *Psychological Bulletin, 139,* 152-188.

7. Ware, J. E., Jr., Snow, K. K., Kosinski, M., & Gnadek, B. (1993). *SF-36 Health Survey: Manual and interpretation guide.* Boston, MA: The Health Institute, New England Medical Center.

**PSYCHE
BOOKS**

The study of the mind: interactions, behaviours, functions.
Developing and learning our understanding of self. Psyche
Books cover all aspects of psychology and matters relating to
the head.